COMLEX Review

Clinical Anatomy and Osteopathic Manipulative Medicine

COMLEX REVIEW

Clinical Anatomy and Osteopathic Manipulative Medicine

Rupen G. Modi, M.B.A.

Pre-doctoral Teaching Fellow
Dept. of Osteopathic
   Manipulative Medicine
New York College of
   Osteopathic Medicine
Old Westbury, NY

Naishadh A. Shah, M.B.A.

Pre-doctoral Teaching Fellow
Department of Anatomy
New York College of
   Osteopathic Medicine
Old Westbury, NY

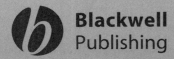
Blackwell Publishing

Blackwell Publishing, Inc., 350 Main Street, Malden, Massachusetts 02148-5018, USA
Blackwell Publishing Ltd, 9600 Garsington Road, Oxford OX4 2DQ, UK
Blackwell Publishing Asia Pty Ltd, 550 Swanston Street, Carlton, Victoria 3053, Australia

05 06 07 08 5 4 3 2 1

ISBN-13: 978-1-4051-0448-7
ISBN-10: 1-4051-0448-1

Library of Congress Cataloging-in-Publication Data

Modi, Rupen G.
   COMLEX review : clinical anatomy and osteopathic manipulative medicine / Rupen G. Modi, Naishadh A. Shah. – 1st ed.
      p. ; cm.
   ISBN-13: 978-1-4051-0448-7 (pbk. : alk. paper)
   ISBN-10: 1-4051-0448-1 (pbk. : alk. paper)
   1. Osteopathic medicine–Examinations, questions, etc. 2. Osteopathic Orthopedics–Examinations, questions, etc. 3. Anatomy–Examinations, questions, etc. I. Shah, Naishadh A. II. Title. III. Title: Clinical anatomy and osteopathic manipulative medicine. [DNLM: 1. Manipulation, Osteopathic–Examination Questions.   2. Anatomy–Examination Questions.   3. Osteopathic Medicine–Examination Questions.   WB 18.2 M692c 2006]
RZ343 .M63 2006
615.5′33′076–dc22

2005010316

A catalogue record for this title is available from the British Library

Acquisitions: Nancy Anastasi Duffy
Development: Selene Steneck
Production: Jennifer Kowalewski
Cover and Interior design: Quantam Corral
Typesetter: SNP Best-set Typesetter Ltd., Hong Kong
Printed and bound by Sheridan Books in Ann Arbor, MI

For further information on Blackwell Publishing, visit our website:
www.blackwellmedstudent.com

Notice: The indications and dosages of all drugs in this book have been recommended in the medical literature and conform to the practices of the general community. The medications described do not necessarily have specific approval by the Food and Drug Administration for use in the diseases and dosages for which they are recommended. The package insert for each drug should be consulted for use and dosage as approved by the FDA. Because standards for usage change, it is advisable to keep abreast of revised recommendations, particularly those concerning new drugs.

The publisher's policy is to use permanent paper from mills that operate a sustainable forestry policy, and which has been manufactured from pulp processed using acid-free and elementary chlorine-free practices. Furthermore, the publisher ensures that the text paper and cover board used have met acceptable environmental accreditation standards.

To my mom and dad—who have taught me about ambition, passion and sacrifice.

To my sister and brother-in-law—who have taught me to work hard and achieve any goal.

To my nieces—who have taught me to always smile.

– R.M.

To my mother, father, and sister who have always made my happiness their number one priority.

To my large family and group of friends who have remained close no matter how far my ambitions have taken me.

And finally, to the teachings of Jainism, which have always guided me to the paths of compassion, tolerance, and education.

– N.S.

CONTENTS

SECTION V: THORACIC, ABDOMINAL, AND PELVIC VISCERA

SECTION VI: OSTEOPATHIC APPROACH TO SPECIALTIES

FACULTY ADVISORS

Claudia L. McCarty, D.O., F.A.A.O.
Private Practice
Osteopathic Manipulative Medicine Associates
Syosset, New York

John P. Hunter, Ph.D.
Department of Evolution, Ecology & Organismal Biology
Ohio State University
Newark, OH

CONTRIBUTORS

Lanna Cheuck
Pre-doctoral Fellow, Dept. of Anatomy
New York College of Osteopathic Medicine
Old Westbury, New York

Jennifer Epperlein
Pre-doctoral Fellow, Dept. of OMM
New York College of Osteopathic Medicine
Old Westbury, New York

Golru Ghaffari
Pre-doctoral Fellow, Dept. of OMM
New York College of Osteopathic Medicine
Old Westbury, New York

Reem Jaber-Iqbal
Pre-doctoral Fellow, Dept. of OMM
New York College of Osteopathic Medicine
Old Westbury, New York

Rachel LaMonica
Pre-doctoral Fellow, Dept. of OMM
New York College of Osteopathic Medicine
Old Westbury, New York

Tara A. McConnon
Pre-doctoral Fellow, Dept. of OMM
New York College of Osteopathic Medicine
Old Westbury, New York

Brian Peter Mieczkowski
Pre-doctoral Fellow, Dept. of Anatomy
New York College of Osteopathic Medicine
Old Westbury, New York

Scott Newsome, DO
Resident, Dept. of Neurology
Albany Medical Center
Albany, New York

Anand Panchal
Pre-doctoral Fellow, Dept. of Anatomy
New York College of Osteopathic Medicine
Old Westbury, New York

Ripal Parikh
Pre-doctoral Fellow, Dept. of OMM
New York College of Osteopathic Medicine
Old Westbury, New York

Sonia Rivera-Martinez, DO
Resident, Dept. of Family Medicine
Long Beach Medical Center
Long Beach, New York

Rosanna C. Sabini
Pre-doctoral Fellow, Dept. of OMM
New York College of Osteopathic Medicine
Old Westbury, New York

Anne Shapiro
Pre-doctoral Fellow, Dept. of Anatomy
New York College of Osteopathic Medicine
Old Westbury, New York

Patricia A. Snyder, DO, MS
Resident, Dept. of Obstetrics and Gynecology
Albany Medical Center
Albany, New York

Matthew Sommella, DO
Resident, Dept. of General Surgery
St. Barnabas Hospital
Bronx, New York

Amy L. Spizuoco
Pre-doctoral Fellow, Dept. of OMM
New York College of Osteopathic Medicine
Old Westbury, New York

Julie A. Sylvester
Pre-doctoral Fellow, Dept. of OMM
New York College of Osteopathic Medicine
Old Westbury, New York

Michael Tamburo
Pre-doctoral Fellow, Dept. of OMM
New York College of Osteopathic Medicine
Old Westbury, New York

Brian M. Walters
Pre-doctoral Fellow, Dept. of OMM
New York College of Osteopathic Medicine
Old Westbury, New York

CONTRIBUTING REVIEWERS

Noeen Ahmad
Medical Student, Class of 2005
New York College of Osteopathic Medicine
Old Westbury, New York

Kelly M. Dease
Pre-doctoral Fellow, Dept. of OMM
New York College of Osteopathic Medicine
Old Westbury, New York

Neha R. Vagadia, DO
Resident, Dept. of Internal Medicine
University of Massachusetts Medical Center
Worcester, Massachusetts

REVIEWERS

Jason Allen
4th year student
Kansas City University of Medicine and Biosciences
Kansas City, Missouri

Suzanne Crandall
4th year student
Kansas City University of Medicine and Biosciences
Kansas City, Missouri

Rachel Dawson, DO
Class of 2004
Nova Southeastern University College of Osteopathic Medicine
Fort Lauderdale, Florida

Amanda Flynn, DO
Class of 2004
Nova Southeastern University College of Osteopathic Medicine
Fort Lauderdale, Florida

Mark Hafen, DO
Class of 2004
Kirksville College of Osteopathic Medicine
Kirksville, Missouri

Jacob Hansen
3rd year student
Kirksville College of Osteopathic Medicine
Kirksville, Missouri

Cathy Sims O'Neil
4th year student
University of New England College of Osteopathic Medicine
Biddeford, Maine

Joey Scafidi, DO
The University Children's Hospital
University of Medicine and Dentistry of New Jersey
Newark, New Jersey

David M. Skeehan, DO
General Surgery Intern
Mount Clemens General Hospital
Mount Clemens, MI

PREFACE

We have tried to make studying for the Comprehensive Osteopathic Medicine Licensing Exam (COMLEX-USA) as pleasant, interactive, and enjoyable as possible. This book will help you to review and recall the high-yield facts about Clinical Anatomy and Osteopathic Manipulative Medicine needed to ensure a score you'll be satisfied with. Instead of presenting random facts and ideas in an outline or paragraph form, you will be able to actively challenge your memory with our question and answer format.

We suggest that you integrate the Gross Anatomy Overview with the Clinical Anatomy and Osteopathic Principles subsections. This book is organized so that you may review anatomy (as a fundamental) before moving on to its clinical applications.

This book has been written with students studying for all three levels of the COMLEX in mind. For ease of use, we have broken the book down into sections that pertain to different levels of training. The following checklist is provided to suggest areas that may prove most useful to readers at specific points in their academic career.

First Year Student	Second Year Student	3rd & 4th Year Student*	Intern*
☐ Section I	☐ Section III	☐ Section IV	☐ Section I
☐ Section II	☐ Section IV	☐ Section VII	☐ Section VI
Anatomy Subsections of:	☐ Section V	☐ Section VI	
☐ Section III	☐ Section VI		
☐ Section IV			
☐ Section V			

Level 1 Examinee	Level 2 Examinee*	Level 3 Examinee*
☐ Section I	☐ Section I	☐ Section I
☐ Section II	☐ Section II	☐ Section II
☐ Section III	☐ Section III	☐ Section III
☐ Section IV	☐ Section IV	☐ Section IV
☐ Anatomy Subsections from Section V	☐ Section V	☐ Section V
	☐ Section VI	☐ Section VI

* You may skim or skip over the Gross Anatomy Overview section.

Additional information about the COMLEX can be obtained from the web site of the National Board of Osteopathic Medical Examiners at http://www.nbome.org.

– Rupen G. Modi and Naishadh A. Shah

We hope that you find *COMLEX Review: Clinical Anatomy and Osteopathic Manipulative Medicine* informative and useful. We welcome feedback and suggestions you have about this book, or any published by Blackwell Publishing.

Please e-mail us at medfeedback@bos.blackwellpublishing.com.

Acknowledgments

We are very grateful to all our professors, attendings, and colleagues who have given us the knowledge, inspiration, and confidence to put this book together. Dr. Claudia L. McCarty and Dr. John P. Hunter were a great asset as our faculty advisors, without whom this book would not be the same. Our contributors and reviewers have helped shape this project in many ways, and we extend our warmest thanks to them as well. The efforts of Blackwell Publishing and the wonderful personalities of individuals such as Nancy Duffy, Selene Steneck, and Susan Burcham complemented our efforts beyond description. Dr. Richard J. Claps and Dr. George T. Veliath deserve special mention for providing the necessary radiographs from Union Hospital, Union, NJ.

We would also like to acknowledge the Deans, the Department of Anatomy, and the Stanley Schiowitz, DO, FAAO, Department of Osteopathic Manipulative Medicine of the New York College of Osteopathic Medicine for their support and encouragement.

We dedicate this book to all the osteopathic medical students that wear their short white coats with pride every day for 4 years, never complaining about hard work or their sacrifices (even though the hospital janitors and cafeteria workers get to wear long coats!).

We would also like to dedicate this book to all the pre-doctoral teaching fellows at the Osteopathic Medical Schools across the country, for their dedication to sharing what they have learned and their energy toward being role model students.

Figure Credits

Figures 1.2a, 1.2b, 8.6 (modified), 11.9, 11.10, 11.11, 11.12, and 11.13 (modified), reproduced with permission from the American Association of the Colleges of Osteopathic Medicine's Glossary of Osteopathic Terminology, 2002.

Figures 3.2, 3.3, 3.5, 3.6, 3.7, 3.8, 3.9, 3.10, 3.11, 3.12, 3.13, 3.14, 3.15, 5.3, 5.4, 5.8, 5.9, 6.5, 7.1, 7.2, 7.4, 7.5, 7.7, 9.8, 10.5, 10.6, 10.8a, 10.8b, 10.9, 11.1a, 11.1b, 11.2, 11.4, 11.8, 12.3, 12.4a, 12.4b, 12.4c, 12.5, 12.10, 12.11a, 12.11b, 12.11c, 13.1, 13.2, 13.3, 13.6a, 13.6b, 13.11a, 13.11b, 13.11c, 13.12, 13.13, 13.14, 13.15, 13.16, 13.17, 13.18, 13.19, and 13.20 reproduced with permission from Ellis H. Clinical Anatomy: A revision and applied anatomy for clinical students. 10th ed. Oxford: Blackwell Science, 2002.

Figures 4.2, 4.3, 6.3a, 6.3b, 6.4, 6.6, 6.7, 8.3, 8.4, 8.5, 11.7, and 12.12 reproduced with permission from Ellis H, Feldman S, Harrop-Griffiths W. Anatomy for Anaesthetists. 8th ed. Oxford: Blackwell Science, 2004.

Figures 4.4, 9.2, and 10.13 reproduced with permission from Gross J, Fetto J, Rosen E. Musculoskeletal Examination. 2nd ed. Malden, MA: Blackwell Science, 2002.

Figures 5.5, 5.6, 9.3, 9.4, 10.2a, 10.2b, 10.2c, 10.2d, 10.2e, 10.3, 11.3, 12.6a, 12.6b, 12.6c, 12.7, 12.8, 12.9, 13.4, 13.5, 13.7a, 13.7b, 13.7c, 13.7d, 13.7e, 13.8a, 13.8b, 13.9, and 13.10 reproduced with permission from Whitaker RH, Borley N. Instant Anatomy. Oxford: Blackwell Science, 2000.

Figures 5.10, 5.11a, 5.11b, and 5.12 reproduced with permission from Digiovanna EL, Schiowitz S, Dowling D. An Osteopathic Approach to Diagnosis and Treatment. 3rd ed. Philadelphia: Lippincott Williams & Wilkins, 2004.

Figures 9.6, 9.7, 10.11, 12.1, 12.2, 23.1, 23.2, 23.3, 23.4, and 23.5 reproduced with permission from Union Hospital, Union, NJ.

♀	female	DM	diabetes mellitus
♂	male	DRE	digital rectal exam
↑/↓	increase/decrease	DTR	deep tendon reflex
a.	artery	DVT	deep vein thrombosis
AA	atlanto-axial	Dx	diagnosis
aa.	arteries	Dysfxn	dysfunction
AC	acromioclavicular	ECG	electrocardiogram
ACE	angiotensin-converting enzyme	ED	emergency department
ACL	anterior cruciate ligament	ER	external rotation
ADH	antidiuretic hormone	ESR	erythrocyte sedimentation rate
AIIS	anterior inferior iliac spine	FDP	flexor digitorum profundus m.
A.K.A.	also known as	FDS	flexor digitorum superficialis (sublimis) m.
ANS	automatic nervous system		
ant.	anterior	FEV$_1$	forced expiratory volume at 1 second
AOA	American Osteopathic Association		
A-P, AP	anteroposterior	FPR	facilitated positional release
ASA	aspirin	FROM	free range of motion
ASCD	atherosclerotic cardiovascular disease	GE	gastroesophageal
		GERD	gastroesophageal reflux disease
ASIS	anterior superior iliac spine	GFR	glomerular filtration rate
ATF	anterior talofibular	GI	gastrointestinal
A-V	arteriovenous	H&P	history & physical
BLT	balanced ligamentous tension	Hb$_{A1C}$	glycosylated hemoglobin
BP	blood pressure	HIV	human immunodeficiency virus
BPH	benign prostatic hypertrophy	HJR	hepatojugular reflex
bpm	beats per minute	HPI	history of present illness
BUN	blood urea nitrogen	HR	heart rate
c/o	complains of	HSM	hepatosplenomegaly
CABG	coronary artery bypass graft	HTN	hypertension
CC	chief complaint	HVLA	high velocity low amplitude
CD	Crohn's disease	IBD	inflammatory bowel disease
CHF	congestive heart failure	IBS	irritable bowel syndrome
CN	cranial nerve	ICU	intensive care unit
C$_o$	coccyx	ILA	inferolateral angle
CO	cardiac output	IM	intramuscular
COPD	chronic obstructive pulmonary disease	IR	internal rotation
		ITB	iliotibial band
CRI	cranial rhythmic impulse	IV	intravenous
CS	counterstrain	IVC	inferior vena cava
CSF	cerebrospinal fluid	IV disc	intervertebral disc
CT	computed tomography	JRA	juvenile rheumatoid arthritis
CXR	chest x-ray	JVD	jugular venous distention
CVA	cerebrovascular accident	LAS	ligamentous articular strain
DIP	distal interphalangeal	LBP	low back pain
DJD	degenerative joint disease	LCL	lateral collateral ligament

LE	lower extremity	r/o	rule out
LES	lower esophageal sphincter	RA	rheumatoid arthritis
LP	lumbar puncture	RCL	radial collateral ligament
LS	lumbosacral	RLQ	right lower quandrant
LV	left ventricle	ROM	range of motion
m.	muscle	ROS	review of systems
mm.	muscles	RTM	reciprocal tension membrane
MCL	medial collateral ligament	RUQ	right upper quadrant
MCP	metacarpophalangeal	SA	sinoatrial (atrial sinus)
ME	muscle energy	SBJ	sphenobasilar junction
MF	myofascial	SBR	sidebending-rotation
MI	myocardial infarction	SBS	sphenobasilar symphysis, synchondrosis
MRI	magnetic resonance imaging		
MTP	metatarsophalangeal	SBU	sacral base unleveling
n.	nerve	SCFE	slipped capital femoral epiphysis
nn.	nerves	SCM	sternocleidomastoid muscle
NPO	nothing by mouth	SD	somatic dysfunction
NRDS	neonatal respiratory distress syndrome	SI	sacroiliac
		SNS	sympathetic nervous system
NSAIDs	nonsteroidal anti-inflammatory drugs	SOAP	subjective, objective, assessment, plan
OCF	osteopathy in the cranial field	SOB	shortness of breath
OM	occipitomastoid	s/p	status post
OMM	osteopathic manipulative medicine	SP	spinous process
OMT	osteopathic manipulative treatment	SV	stroke volume
		SVC	superior vena cava
OTC	over-the-counter	SVT	supraventricular tachycardia
PCL	posterior cruciate ligament	TM	tympanic membrane
PEEP	positive end-expiratory pressure	TMJ	temporomandibular joint
PFT	pulmonary function test	TOC	test of choice
PIIS	posterior inferior iliac spine	TP	transverse process
PIP	proximal interphalangeal	TPR	total peripheral resistance
PMH/PMHx	past medical history	TRH	thyrotropin-releasing hormone
PMI	point of maximal impulse (heart)	TSH	thyroid-stimulating hormone
PMS	premenstrual syndrome	TURP	transurethral resection of the prostate
PNS	parasympathetic nervous system		
post.	posterior	TV	tidal volume
PRM	primary respiratory mechanism	Tx	treatment
PSH/PSHx	past surgical history	UC	ulcerative colitis
PSIS	posterior superior iliac spine	UCL	ulnar collateral ligament
pt	patient	UE	upper extremity
PTF	posterior talofibular ligament	UMN	upper motor neuron
PTU	propylthiouracil	UPJ	uteropelvic junction
PUD	peptic ulcer disease	URI	upper respiratory infection
PUV	posterior urethral valves	US	ultrasound
PVM	paravertebral muscles	UTI	urinary tract infection
PVMS	paravertebral muscle spasm	UVJ	uterovesicular junction

v.	vein	VT	ventricular tachycardias
VMO	vastus medialis obliqus m.	vv.	veins
V/Q	ventilation-to-perfusion ratio	XR	x-ray

SECTION I

Osteopathic Practices and Principles

BASIC PRINCIPLES

What are the four basic principles of osteopathic medicine?

1. **The body is a unit.**
2. **The body is self-regulating and self-healing.**
3. **Structure and function are reciprocally related.**
4. **Rational treatment is based on this philosophy and these principles.**

What is the somatic system?

It is the body framework involving the skeletal, arthrodial, and myofascial structures, and their related vascular, lymphatic, and neural elements.

What is a somatic dysfunction?

Impaired or altered function of related components of the somatic (body framework) system.

What are the four basic characteristics of a somatic dysfunction on exam?

<u>1.</u> <u>T</u>issue texture changes
<u>2.</u> <u>A</u>symmetry
<u>3.</u> <u>R</u>estriction of motion
<u>4.</u> <u>T</u>enderness (or <u>S</u>ensitivity changes)

 Memory Aid: **TART** or **STAR**

TABLE 1.1 – **Acute versus Chronic Somatic Dysfunctions**

Characteristic	Acute SD	Chronic SD
Range of motion	Restricted	Restricted
Tenderness	Sharp (more tender than chronic SD)	Dullness and paresthesia
Erythema	Present Apparent with erythema (red reflex) test	Pale Immediate blanching following erythema test
Skin temperature	Warm	Cool
Skin moisture	Increased Apparent with increased skin drag	Decreased (dry)
Muscle and soft tissue	Boggy, edematous, increased muscle tone	Ropy, fibrotic, decreased muscle tone

SD, somatic dysfunction.

How are somatic dysfunctions named?	Somatic dysfunction nomenclature is based upon the freedom of motion.
Define the following types of barriers:	
Physiologic barrier	**The limitation of active range of motion (ROM) in the absence of any pathologic process.**
Anatomic barrier	**The limitation of passive ROM in the absence of any pathologic process. This ROM is generally greater than physiologic barrier.**
Pathologic barrier	The limitation of physiologic and/or anatomic ROM as a result of a disease process.
Osteopathic restrictive barrier	**A type of pathologic barrier restricting physiologic ROM and resulting in asymmetry of this motion (somatic dysfunction).**
What is a somato-somatic reflex?	**A somatic dysfunction produces a stimulus that may generate a secondary somatic dysfunction elsewhere.**
What is a somato-visceral reflex?	A somatic dysfunction produces a stimulus that may generate a dysfunction of the visceral (organ) system.
What is a viscero-visceral reflex?	A dysfunction of the visceral system produces a stimulus that may generate a secondary visceral dysfunction elsewhere.
What is a viscero-somatic reflex?	**A dysfunction of the visceral system produces a stimulus that may generate a somatic dysfunction.**
What is facilitation?	A dysfunction can decrease the threshold for excitation of neurons innervating the region of dysfunction. This lowered threshold of neurons is facilitation. Facilitation may lead to dysfunctions in regions innervated by the same pool of neurons.

Autonomic nervous system innervation (Table 1.2)

TABLE 1.2 – **Autonomic Nervous System**

Organ	Sympathetic Innervation (spinal cord segments)	Parasympathetic Innervation (spinal cord segments and cranial nerves)
Head and neck	T1–T4	Cranial nerves (III, VII, IX, X)
Trachea and bronchi	T1–T5	Vagus n.
Esophagus (distal ⅔)	T1 or T2–T6 or T8	Vagus n.
Lung parenchyma	T1–T6	Vagus n.
Lung visceral pleura	T1–T7	Vagus n.
Lung parietal pleura	T1–T11	Vagus n.
Heart	T1–T5 or T6	Vagus n.
Stomach and duodenum (proximal)	T5–T9	Vagus n.
Intestinal tract	T5–L2	Vagus n. and sacral plexus
Midgut—duodenum (distal), jejunum, ileum, appendix, ascending colon and transverse colon (proximal ⅔)	T10–T11 or T12	Vagus n.
Hindgut—transverse colon (distal ⅓), descending colon, sigmoid colon, and rectum	T12–L2	S2–S4
Appendix	T10 or T12 (right)	Vagus n.
Liver	T5–T9	Vagus n.
Gallbladder and ducts	T5–T7 (right)	Vagus n. (right/posterior)
Pancreas	T7	Vagus n.
Spleen	T7 (left)	Vagus n. (left/posterior)
Adrenal glands	T10–T11	None
Kidneys	T10–T11	Vagus n.
Proximal ureters	T10–T11 or T12	Vagus n.
Distal ureters	T12–L1 or L1–L2	S2–S4
Urinary bladder and urethra	T12–L2	S2–S4
Prostate or uterus/cervix	T10 or T12–L2	S2–S4
Testes or ovaries	T10–T11	S2–S4
Penis or clitoris	T12–L2	S2–S4
Upper extremity	T1 or T2–T8	None
Lower extremity	T10 or T11–L2	None

FRYETTE'S PRINCIPLES

What are Fryette's Principles?	Description of the physiologic motion of the thoracic and lumbar spine.
What is Fryette's First Principles?	**When the thoracic and lumbar spine is in the neutral position, the coupled motions of sidebending and rotation for a group of vertebrae are such that sidebending and rotation occur in opposite directions.**
What is Fryette's Second Principles?	**When the thoracic and lumbar spine is sufficiently forward or backward bent (non-neutral), the coupled motions of sidebending and rotation in a single vertebral unit occur in the same direction.**
What is Fryette's Third Principles?	**Initiating motion of a vertebral segment in any plane of motion will modify the movement of that segment in other planes of motion.**
What is a type I somatic dysfunction?	A group curve of thoracic and/or lumbar vertebrae in which the freedoms of motion are in neutral with sidebending and rotation in opposite directions. The maximum rotation is found at the apical vertebra based on the first principle of Fryette.
What are group curves?	Three or more consecutive thoracic and/or lumbar vertebrae with type I somatic dysfunctions.
In a group curve, what is the relationship between the side of the convexity to the side of sidebending and rotation?	Rotation occurs toward the convexity. Sidebending occurs opposite to the convexity (toward the concavity).
What is the difference between the normal motion of the thoracic/lumbar vertebrae and the motion of type I somatic dysfunctions?	When sitting upright, the asymmetry of sidebending/rotation corrects in normal vertebrae. Whereas, in type I somatic dysfunctions, the asymmetry persists.
What is a type II somatic dysfunction?	Thoracic or lumbar somatic dysfunction of a single vertebral unit in which the vertebra is significantly flexed or extended with sidebending and rotation in the same direction based on the second principle of Fryette.

BASICS OF OSTEOPATHIC MANIPULATIVE TREATMENT

Define the following:

Active motion	Any motion created by one's own muscle contraction.
Passive motion	Any motion induced by an external force without one's own muscle contraction.
Isokinetic resistance	**The resistance applied to a motion allowing movement at a constant speed.**
Isometric resistance	**The resistance applied to a motion preventing any movement while sustaining a constant muscle contraction.**
Active treatment	Patient-assisted treatment therapies (in the form of voluntary contraction and movement).
Passive treatment	Treatment without any voluntary patient assistance.
Direct treatment*	Treatment in which the restrictive barrier(s) is engaged. These techniques involve movement **directly through the restrictive barrier**.
Indirect treatment*	Treatment in which movement is **away from the restrictive barrier**. Movement is in the direction of freedom to **indirectly** treat the restriction.

* Definitions do not apply to direct/indirect active myofascial release techniques.

Classification of techniques (Table 1.3)

TABLE 1.3 – **Classification of Techniques**

	Active	Passive
Direct	Muscle Energy Myofascial	HVLA (and other articulatory techniques) BLT LAS Myofascial OCF Lymphatic treatment Chapman's reflexes
Indirect	Myofascial	Counterstrain FPR BLT LAS Myofascial OCF

HVLA, high velocity low amplitude; BLT, balanced ligamentous tension; LAS, ligamentous articular strain; OCF, osteopathy in the cranial field; FPR, facilitated positional release.

What are the goals of treatment using osteopathic manipulation?

1. Decrease muscle contraction
2. Increase blood/oxygen supply
3. Increase venous and lymphatic drainage
4. Stimulate hypotonic muscles

MYOFASCIAL TECHNIQUES

Define myofascial (MF) techniques.	A soft tissue technique directed toward muscles (myo-) and fascia.
What are the different types of MF techniques?	1. Passive MF 2. Active direct MF 3. Active indirect MF
What are the common indications for MF?	↑ muscle spasm/tension and ↓ vascular/lymphatic flow. Preparation for high velocity low amplitude.
List common contraindications for MF.	Fracture, open wound, or infection.

COUNTERSTRAIN

What is counterstrain (CS)?	A passive, indirect technique using the neuromuscular basis of somatic dysfunction. The body is positioned at a point of ease and balance by straining a muscle at a joint and shortening its antagonist to relieve pain.
Define "tenderpoints."	**Small (~1 cm) fibrotic, edematous areas that are painful to palpation. They are typically found in muscle bellies, ligaments, or tendons.**
What is a "mobile point?"	**A specific position of ease and balance where pain is reduced/relieved at the tenderpoint.**
Describe the physiologic basis for CS.	**Successful CS treatment resets the muscle spindle reflex. The muscle spindle is a mechanoreceptor responsible for detecting muscle load/stretch.**
Define "Travell's (MF) trigger points."	A hypersensitive center found in taut skeletal muscle and fascia, which can present as a consistent referred pain pattern.
What are the common indications for CS?	↑ muscle spasm/tension and ↓ vascular/lymphatic flow.
List common contraindications for CS.	Fracture, open wound, or infection.

MUSCLE ENERGY TECHNIQUES

Define muscle energy (ME).	An active, direct treatment involving voluntary and precise patient movement against isometric resistance away from a pathologic barrier engaged by the physician.
Describe the physiologic basis for ME.	**Successful ME treatment results in reflexive relaxation of agonist muscle fibers. The isometric resistance resets the Golgi tendon organ sensation of the induced tension.**
What are the common indications for ME?	Muscular or joint restrictions.
List common contraindications for ME.	Fracture or torn muscle. Post-surgical and ICU patients.

FACILITATED POSITIONAL RELEASE

Define facilitated positional release (FPR).	A passive, indirect technique in which tissue and joint tension is first neutralized (diminished) followed by compression (an activating force) and then addition of freedom of motion in side-bending and rotation. It is derived from CS.
What are the three steps of FPR?	**1. Neutral positioning** **2. Facilitating motion (compression or torsion)** **3. Move toward freedom (indirect position)**
Describe the physiologic basis for FPR.	Successful FPR treatment resets the muscle spindle reflex (similar to CS).
What are the common indications for FPR?	Hypertonic muscles (superficial or deep) and somatic dysfunctions (type I and type II).
List common contraindications for FPR.	Fracture, open wound, or infection.

HIGH VELOCITY LOW AMPLITUDE

Define high velocity low amplitude (HVLA).	A passive, direct treatment where the physician engages the pathologic barrier and uses a precise, quick, and small thrust through the restrictive barrier.
What are the common indications for HVLA?	↓ ROM. HVLA is more advantageous when the barrier is firm.

9

List the common absolute and relative contraindications for HVLA.

Absolute: osteoporosis, osteopenia, osteomyelitis, fracture, dislocation, skeletal neoplasm, severe rheumatoid arthritis (especially cervical HVLA), Down's syndrome.

Relative: blood dyscrasia, pneumonia, coagulopathy/anticoagulation, acute muscle injury, acute whiplash, neurologic pathologies/radiculopathies, herniated intervertebral discs, vertebral arterial stenosis, cerebrovascular accident, pregnancy, open wounds, recent surgery, hypermobile joints.

LIGAMENTOUS ARTICULAR STRAIN/BALANCED LIGAMENTOUS TENSION

Define ligamentous articular strain (LAS).

A passive technique for the treatment of somatic dysfunction across joints by balancing ligamentous tension.

What is another name for LAS?

Balanced ligamentous tension.

What are the common indications for LAS?

Somatic dysfunctions of ligaments across joints and sprains.

List common contraindications for LAS.

Fracture, torn muscle.

CHAPMAN'S REFLEXES

What are Chapman's points?

Small (2–3 mm), firm, gangliform contractions resulting from ↑ congestion and ↑ sympathetic tone due to lymphatic edema/myofascial thickening. (See Figures 1.1A and 1.1B.)

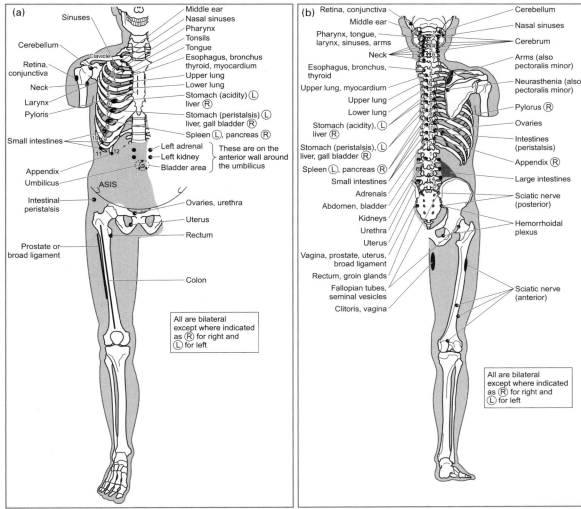

FIGURE I.IA – Anterior Chapman's points.

FIGURE I.IB – Posterior Chapman's points.

What type of reflex is the Chapman's reflex?	**Viscerosomatic reflex.**
How are Chapman's points treated?	Applying gentle circular pressure over the point until the nodule dissipates.
What are the common indications for Chapman's point treatment?	↑ muscle spasm/tension and ↓ vascular/lymphatic flow.
List common contraindications for Chapman's point treatment.	Fracture, open wound, or infection.

LYMPHATIC TECHNIQUES

What autonomic nervous system innervates the lymphatic system?	Sympathetic nervous system. Increased sympathetic tone may cause the lymphatic vessels to constrict and lead to decreased lymphatic return and edema distally.
What factors promote lymphatic flow?	**Respiration, vascular blood flow, muscle contractions, body movement.**
Lymph from what structures drain into the right lymphatic duct?	**Right hemicranium, right face, right upper extremity, right breast, heart and all lobes of the lungs except the left upper lobe.**
What is necessary before performing any lymphatic treatment?	**Release of all diaphragms en route for lymph return to the thoracic duct.**
What are the indications for lymphatic treatment?	Upper respiratory infection, bronchitis, pneumonia, asthma, chronic obstructive pulmonary disease, atelactasis, s/p myocardial infarction, congestive heart failure, endocarditis, mastitis, lymphedema, inflammatory bowel disease, chronic hepatitis, cirrhosis, pancreatitis, nephrotic syndrome, premenstrual syndrome, uterine fibroid, endometriosis, cystitis, tendonitis, osteomyelitis, eczema, psoriasis, trauma.
List the major contraindications to lymphatic treatment.	Fractures, severe infections (temperature >102°F), abscess, carcinoma.* * *The contraindication to lymphatic treatment in carcinoma is controversial.*

ZINK (COMMON COMPENSATORY) PATTERNS

Where are the four compensatory curves of the axial skeleton located?	1. **Occipito-atlantal junction (OA)** 2. **Cervicothoracic junction (CT)** 3. **Thoracolumbar junction (TL)** 4. **Lumbosacral junction (LS)**

What is the common compensatory pattern described by Zink?

In 80% of healthy individuals, an alternating pattern beginning with the OA rotated left, CT rotated right, TL rotated left, and LS rotated right (see Figure 1.2A).

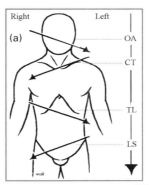

FIGURE 1.2A – Common compensatory pattern of Zink.

What is the uncommon compensatory pattern described by Zink?

In the remaining 20% of healthy individuals, an alternating pattern beginning with the OA rotated right, CT rotated left, TL rotated right, and LS rotated left (see Figure 1.2B).

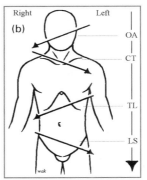

FIGURE 1.2B – Uncommon compensatory pattern of Zink.

What is the significance of the alternating fascial patterns at the transitional junctions of the axial skeleton?

The alternating pattern is necessary for normal lymphatic flow in the body.

What are the results of a disruption in the alternating pattern?

When these patterns are disrupted, illness may ensue. Trauma and stress are possible causes for disruption of the fascial patterns.

2 NOTE WRITING

HISTORY AND PHYSICAL

What is the purpose of a history and physical (H&P)?	To introduce a new patient to any healthcare provider emphasizing all complaints and findings (past and present).

History:

Identification	Name, age, gender, referring physician, and the informant (include reliability of informant).
Chief Complaint (CC)	A brief statement describing the reason the patient is seeking healthcare (generally in the patient's own words).
History of Present Illness (HPI)	This includes further details of the CC. Details such as onset, pain, quality, radiation, severity, timing, setting, frequency, aggravating/alleviating factors, and relevant medical history.
Past Medical History (PMH or PMHx)	Includes information on date and status of all chronic and acute medical illnesses, hospitalizations, ED visits, trauma, blood transfusions, etc.
Past Surgical History (PSH or PSHx)	Includes information on date and complications of all surgeries (same day, inpatient, emergency, trauma, dental, etc.) Do not forget to ask about appendectomy, cholecystectomy, circumcision, cesarean section, and tonsillectomy.
Medications (Meds)/Treatments	Information on dates and satisfaction with past and current medications (prescribed/over-the-counter/herbal/vitamins) and OMT.
Allergies	Information on environmental, drug and food allergies/adverse reactions. Include description, severity, and treatment details for each reaction.
Family History	Include age, status (alive, deceased) and medical problems of blood relatives.

Social History	Marital status; employment history; tobacco, alcohol, and drug use; diet; stressors; lifestyle risk factors; children; education; religion; sexual practices; sleep patterns; etc.
Review of Systems (ROS)	A brief description of the patient's other complaints, concerns, or observations in the following body systems: skin, head, eyes, ears, nose, mouth/throat, neck, respiratory, cardiovascular, breast/chest, gastrointestinal, genitourinary, ob/gyn, musculoskeletal, endocrine, neuropsychiatric, general, etc.

Physical Exam:

Vitals	Temperature, pulse, respiratory rate, blood pressure, O_2 saturation.
General	Description of the patient's attitude and appearance. Include mood, development, race, signs of distress, gait, posture, pallor, and body habitus.
Skin	Scars, rashes, eruptions, tattoos, moles, color changes, nails, hair patterns, tissue texture changes, erythema, skin tags, blanching, temperature, moisture/dryness, etc.
Lymph Nodes	Consistency, location, tenderness, size, mobility.
Head	Size, shape, tenderness, bruising, signs of trauma, scars, cranial rhythmic impulse, somatic dysfunctions of the sphenobasilar synchondrosis and occipito-atlantal, motion of cranial and facial bones, temporomandibular joint motion, lymph nodes.
Eyes	Visual acuity, visual fields, conjunctiva, pupil size, pupil reactivity, extraocular muscle movement, fundi, hemorrhages, exudates, A-V nicks (ratios), symmetry of orbits.
Ears	Test hearing, tenderness, discharge, external canal, tympanic membrane, mucous, symmetry of external ear, foreign bodies.
Nose	Anatomic symmetry, discharge, erythema, turbinates, septum, obstruction, lesion. Palpation over frontal, ethmoid, and maxillary sinuses.
Throat/Mouth	Mucous membranes, erythema, discharge, lesions, foreign bodies, tonsils, tongue, gums, lips, teeth, hygiene.
Neck	Lymph nodes, jugular venous distention, range of motion (ROM), thyroid, sternocleidomastoid, strap muscles, bruits, hepato-jugular reflex, Brudzinski's sign, cervical somatic dysfunction(s). Position/mobility of trachea, larynx, and hyoid.

15

Chest/Thorax	Symmetry, shape (e.g., pigeon/barrel), tenderness, motion with respiration, intercostal retractions, tactile fremitus, percussion, whispered pectoriloquy, point of maximal impulse, thymus, somatic dysfunction (thoracic vertebra, ribs, sternum, thoracic inlet).
Lungs	Auscultation (bilateral, apexes and bases), consolidation, bronchophony, egophony, adventitious sounds, breath sounds, transmitted sounds, Hamman's sign (mediastinal crunch).
Heart	Auscultation (aortic, pulmonic, mitral, tricuspid, and Erb's points), rate, S_1, S_2, S_3, S_4, murmurs, gallops, rubs, thrills, clicks, distant/dampened/muffled sounds.
Breast	Symmetry, nipple discharge, color changes, inversion, fissures, dimpling, contour, palpation for mass, tenderness, gynecomastia in males.
Abdomen/Lower Back	Motion with respiration, scars, fat distribution, costal margins, distention, bruits, softness, tenderness, costovertebral/flank pain, somatic dysfunction (lumbar vertebra, diaphragm, ganglions, paravertebral muscles, mesentery). Palpate kidneys and aorta. Bowel sounds, rebound tenderness. Palpate liver, spleen, and ascending/descending/sigmoid colon. Murphy's, psoas, and obturator signs. Scratch test for hepatosplenomegaly.
Pelvic/Rectal	Somatic dysfunction of innominates, sacrum, and associated muscles/pelvic diaphragm. Genitalia appropriate for gender/age, genital lesions, kidney/bladder palpation. For women: bimanual exam, Pap smear, adnexal palpation, vaginal discharge/odor. For men: testicular exam, scrotal swelling, prostate exam, circumcision. Digital rectal exam, hemorrhoids, fissures, abscess, fistulas, guaiac test.
Structural/Musculoskeletal	Symmetry of eyes, ears, shoulders, fingers, iliac crests, gluteal creases, popliteal creases, malleoli, and plantar arches. Vertical alignment from a lateral view of the external auditory canal, humeral head, greater trochanter, and lateral malleolus. Observe changes in cervical lordosis, thoracic kyphosis, and lumbar lordosis. From a posterior view, observe any cervical, thoracic, and lumbar scoliotic curves and/or rib humps. ROM of all joints. Note any swelling, tenderness, warmth, and crepitus at joints. Also note any amputations or deformities.

Extremities	Clubbing, cyanosis, edema, tenderness, peripheral pulses, capillary refill, trauma, lesions, and ROM.
	Upper extremity (UE): Motion of clavicle, scapula, glenohumeral joint, elbow joint, radial head, carpal, metacarpal, and phalanges. Note any muscle spasms and soft-tissue contractures. Apley scratch test, Phalen's test, Tinel's sign, Yergason's test, Allen test, Finkelstein test, arm-drop test, and apprehension test.
	Lower extremity (LE): Motion of hip joint, knee, fibular head, ankle, tarsal bones, metatarsals, phalanges. Note any muscle spasms and soft-tissue contractures. Kernig's, Thomas', Homans, Trendelenburg, Edward's, Thompson tests.
Psychiatric	Appearance, mood, affect, speech, thought process/content, and motor behavior.
Neurologic	CN I–XII, motor (graded strength of UE/LE), deep tendon reflexes, cerebellum (Romberg's test, heel-to-shin, dysdiadochokinesis, etc.), sensory (pain, temperature, vibration, touch, etc.).
Laboratory/Radiology	Include all laboratory results, radiologic studies, ECGs, and pending tests/studies.
Assessment/Impression	Generally a single statement summarizing/listing the current diagnoses and status of a patient. May also include a discussion of the patient's working diagnosis or differential diagnosis.
Plan	Includes any treatments, medications, diagnostic tests, consultations/referrals, patient education, exercises, and/or follow-up.

SOAP NOTE

What is a SOAP Note?	An update (at least daily for in-patients) that emphasizes a patient's progress through their treatment course.
Subjective	"What the patient says." All information collected from patient and other people. Synonymous with chief complaint. Include any improvement/deterioration/ change in symptoms, lab results, studies, diagnosis that you obtain from the patient. Ask patient about impact/effectiveness of treatment/OMT.
Objective	Description of *your* physical findings and recording of diagnostics. Important information to include are vital signs, general appearance, (focused) physical/ structural examination, laboratory data, imaging studies, ancillary tests, and pending data.
Assessment/**P**lan	Same as H&P above.

17

SECTION II

Axial Skeleton

CERVICAL

GROSS ANATOMY OVERVIEW

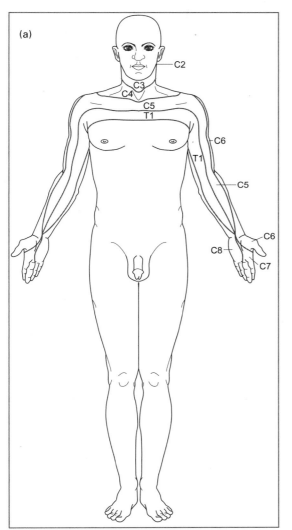
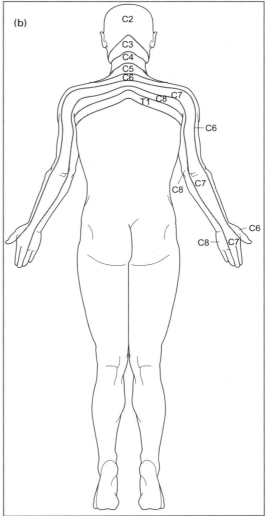

FIGURE 3.1 – Dermatomes from the cervical spine.

What is the primary curvature of the cervical spine?	Lordosis.
How many cervical vertebrae are there? How many cervical spinal nerves exist?	Seven vertebrae (C_1–C_7), but eight cervical spinal nerves exist.
Which cervical spinal nerves exit the intervertebral foramina above their corresponding vertebrae?	Cervical spinal nerves 1 through 7. (C8 exits between C_7 and T_1 vertebrae.)
List the other names for the following vertebrae: C_1. C_2. C_7.	Atlas, axis, and vertebra prominens, respectively.

(💮) *Memory Aid:* These named vertebra are in alphabetical order.

Which cervical vertebra lacks a spinous process and vertebral body?	The atlas (see Figure 3.2).

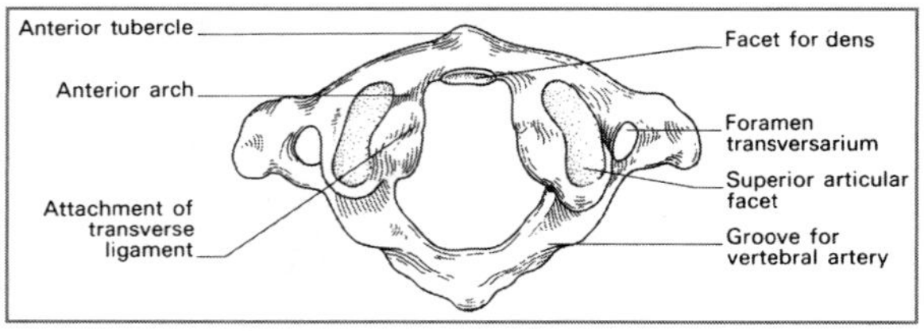

FIGURE 3.2 – C_1 – Atlas.

Name the bony structure that extends from the body of C_2 to articulate with C_1 superiorly.	The dens (A.K.A. odontoid process) (see Figure 3.3).

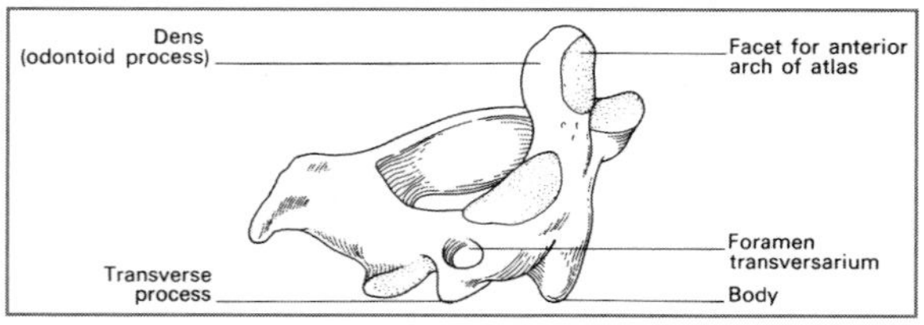

FIGURE 3.3 – C_2 – Axis.

What is a distinguishing feature of the cervical spinous processes?	They are often bifid spinous processes.
How does one vertebra articulate with the vertebrae above and below?	Via the superior and inferior articular facets.
What are two components of an intervertebral disc?	Anulus fibrosus (outer circumference) and nucleus pulposus (center).
What structure courses through the foramen transversarium of most cervical vertebrae?	Vertebral artery.

Which cervical vertebra does not have the vertebral artery coursing through a foramen transversarium?

C_7

Identify the following structures (Figure 3.4):

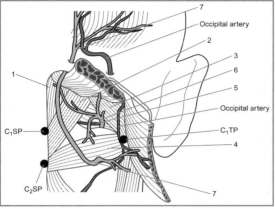

FIGURE 3.4 – Suboccipital triangle.

1. Rectus capitis posterior minor m.
2. Rectus capitis posterior major m.
3. Obliquus capitis superior m.
4. Obliquus capitis inferior m.
5. Vertebral a.
6. Suboccipital n. (dorsal ramus of C1)
7. Greater occipital n. (dorsal ramus of C2)

What is the joint of Luschka (A.K.A. unciform joints)?

The articulation between the vertebral body of a cervical vertebra and the uncinate process of the vertebra below it.

What is the purpose of the joint of Luschka?

To prevent lateral translation of the vertebral bodies relative to each other while allowing for flexion/extension.

List the vertebral levels that correspond to the surface anatomy in Figure 3.5.

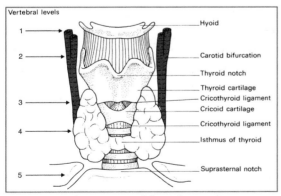

FIGURE 3.5 – Surface anatomy of the neck.

1. C_3
2. C_4
3. C_5
4. C_6
5. T_2

Identify the fascial layers of the neck (Figure 3.6):

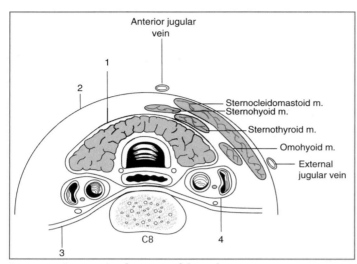

FIGURE 3.6 – Cross-sectional anatomy of the neck.

1. Pretracheal fascia
2. Investing fascia
3. Prevertebral fascia
4. Carotid sheath

What are the contents of the triangles of the neck?
(Figure 3.7)

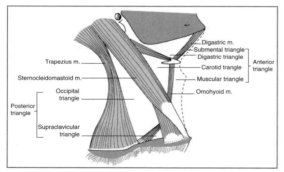

FIGURE 3.7 – Triangles of the neck.

Anterior triangle

- Submandibular (digastric) triangle: hypoglossal n., mylohyoid n., submandibular gland
- Submental triangle: small veins that will form the anterior jugular v.
- Carotid triangle: carotid sheath, hypoglossal n., superior root of ansa cervicalis, CN XI, thyroid, larynx
- Muscular triangle: strap muscles, thyroid and parathyroid

Posterior triangle

- Occipital triangle: external jugular v., CN XI, trunks of brachial plexus
- Supraclavicular triangle: subclavian a. and v., suprascapular a.

What are the actions of the following muscles on the cervical spine:

Anterior, middle, and posterior scalene mm.	Accessory mm. of inspiration. Ipsilateral sidebending of neck.
Sternocleidomastoid (SCM) m.	Ipsilateral sidebending and contralateral rotation. Also accessory m. of inspiration.
Trapezius m.	Extends and sidebends the cervical spine.

What are the contents of the carotid sheath? How are they situated within the sheath?

<u>V</u>agus n. (posterior), <u>I</u>nternal jugular v. (medial), and <u>C</u>arotid a. (lateral).

 Memory Aid: <u>VIC</u> lives in the carotid sheath.

Identify the branches of the external carotid a. (Figure 3.8):

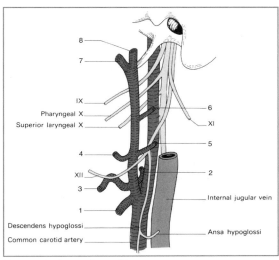

FIGURE 3.8 – External carotid artery.

1. <u>S</u>uperior thyroid a.
2. <u>A</u>scending pharyngeal a.
3. <u>L</u>ingual a.
4. <u>F</u>acial a.
5. <u>O</u>ccipital a.
6. <u>P</u>osterior auricular a.
7. <u>M</u>axillary a.
8. <u>S</u>uperficial temporal a.

 Memory Aid: <u>S</u>even <u>A</u>rtsy <u>L</u>adies <u>F</u>awn <u>O</u>ver <u>P</u>icaso's <u>M</u>arble <u>S</u>culpture.

What is the major blood supply to the thyroid gland?

Superior thyroid a. and inferior thyroid a. (Figure 3.9).

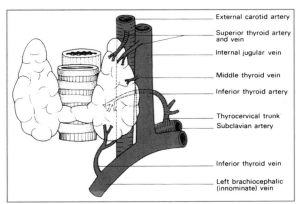

FIGURE 3.9 – Thyroid gland vasculature.

What is the major blood supply to the parathyroid glands?

Inferior thyroid a.

 Memory Aid: The parathyroid glands are smaller than the thyroid, thus the inferior artery supplies them.

Cervical Sympathetic Trunk (Figure 3.10)

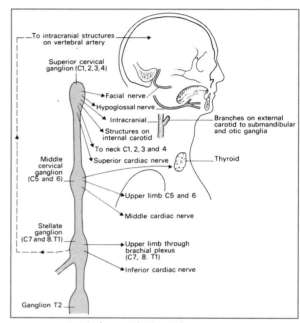

FIGURE 3.10 – Cervical sympathetic trunk.

What nerve innervates the abdominal diaphragm?

The phrenic nerve (arising from nerve roots C3, C4, and C5).

 Memory Aid: C3, C4, and C5 keep the diaphragm alive.

Lymph Nodes of the Neck (Figure 3.11)

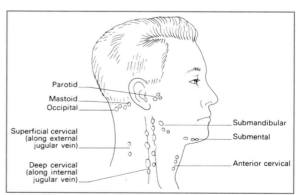

FIGURE 3.11 – Lymph nodes of the neck.

Identify the following structures on the larynx (Figure 3.12):

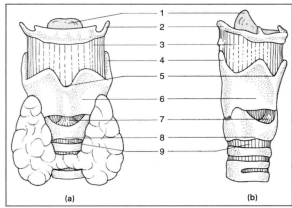

FIGURE 3.12 – Osteology of the larynx.

1. Epiglottis
2. Hyoid
3. Thyrohyoid membrane
4. Superior horn of thyroid cartilage
5. Thyroid notch
6. Body of thyroid cartilage
7. Cricothyroid ligament
8. Cricoid cartilage (ring)
9. Cricotracheal membrane

Internal Structures of the Larynx (Lamina of the thyroid cartilage has been cut away) (Figure 3.13)

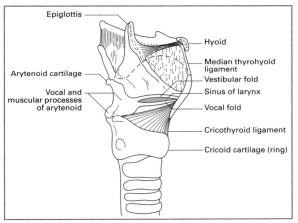

FIGURE 3.13 – Internal structures of the larynx (lamina of the thyroid cartilage has been cut away).

Identify the muscles of the pharynx (see Figure 3.14):

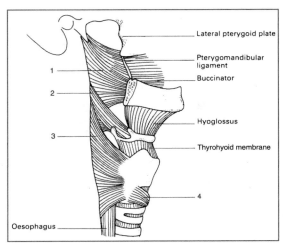

FIGURE 3.14 – Muscles of the pharynx.

1. Superior constrictor m.
2. Middle constrictor m.
3. Inferior constrictor m.
4. Cricothyroid m.

What does the superior laryngeal n. innervate?	Internal branch: pierces thyrohyoid membrane (with superior laryngeal vessels) to supply mucosa of larynx above vocal cords.
	External branch: cricothyroid m.
What innervates the laryngeal mucosa below the vocal cords?	The recurrent laryngeal n. innervates the mucosa below the vocal cords and all intrinsic laryngeal mm. except cricothyroid m.
Which cervical ligaments prevent hyperflexion? Hyperextension? Excessive sidebending?	Hyperflexion: (generally posterior ligaments) Ligamentum nuchae, ligamentum flava, posterior longitudinal ligament, interspinous ligament, and intertransverse ligaments.
	Hyperextension: Anterior longitudinal ligament and intertransverserii ligaments.
	Excessive sidebending: intertransverserii ligaments. *(See Chapter 4: Thoracic, Figure 4.3 Vertebral Ligaments.)*

CLINICAL ANATOMY

What is a Hangman's fracture?	Fracture through the pedicles of the axis (with or without subluxation of the axis on C_3 vertebra). This injury can cause spinal cord lesion resulting in quadriplegia or death.
	Memory Aid: If a "man" were "hanged" from his neck, he would have a fracture in his cervical vertebra.
Where on the trachea is an opening created during a tracheostomy?	Between the first and second tracheal rings or through the second to fourth tracheal rings.
How can an infection of the fascia of the neck spread to the superior mediastinum?	Inferior spread through the retropharyngeal space.
A lesion of the SCM from a traumatic or breech delivery results in what disease process?	**Tort**icollis: the neck is sidebent to affected side while the face is rotated to the opposite direction.
	Memory Aid: A **tortoise** has a stiff neck.

When attempting subclavian vein puncture for central line placement via the infraclavicular approach, what major structures must the physician be sure to avoid puncturing?

Subclavian a., brachial plexus, and parietal pleura (lung).

What symptoms result from a lesion of the sympathetic trunk in the neck?

Horner's syndrome: pupillary constriction, ptosis, vasodilation, and absence of sweating.

 Memory Aid: PAM—"Ptosis, Anhydrosis, and Miosis."

When performing a thyroidectomy, what structures should the surgeon avoid injuring?

Superior and inferior thyroid aa. & vv., superior laryngeal nn., recurrent laryngeal nn., and the parathyroid glands.

What is a thyroglossal duct cyst?

The presence of thyroid tissue anywhere along the path of descent of the developing thyroid gland. Most commonly, this tissue can be found in the foramen cecum of the tongue (Figure 3.15).

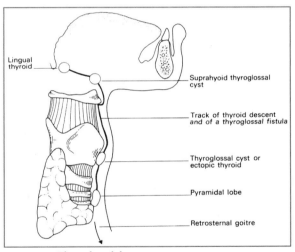

FIGURE 3.15 – Thyroglossal duct cysts.

What are common signs of injury to the recurrent laryngeal n.?

Hoarseness, temporary aphonia, and laryngeal spasm.

Which cervical ligaments are compromised in a patient with whiplash?

Anterior longitudinal ligament, posterior longitudinal ligament, ligamentum nuchae, and intertransverserii ligaments.

What degenerative changes in the cervical spine can result in peripheral neurologic deficits?

Cervical spinal stenosis.

List the major causes of spinal stenosis.	• Congenital • Spondylolisthesis • Osteophytes (i.e., rheumatic conditions) • Disc prolapse

OSTEOPATHIC PRINCIPLES

How is vertebral sidebending (lateral flexion) and translation (lateral slide) coupled?	**Vertebral sidebending to one side is coupled with translation to the opposite side.**
Which vertebra are typical cervical vertebrae?	C_3 to C_7.
What are the characteristics of typical cervical vertebrae?	1. They have vertebral bodies. 2. They articulate at the facets forming articular pillars. 3. They have joints of Luschka.
What motions do the typical cervical vertebrae and C_2 exhibit?	1. Flexion/extension 2. Sidebending/lateral flexion 3. Rotation Note: For purposes of examination, sidebending and rotation of the cervical spine have traditionally been considered to be a coupled motion in the same direction. A 2002 study done by Capobianco and colleagues showed that sidebending and rotation may also occur in opposite directions.
What motions are exhibited at the occipito-atlanto (OA) joint?	1. Flexion/extension 2. Sidebending 3. Rotation Sidebending and rotation at the OA occur in opposite directions.
Why is rotation and sidebending at the OA joint in opposite directions?	Upon rotation at the OA joint, the lateral atlanto-occipital ligament causes the occiput to translate to the same side as the rotation, thus leading to contralateral sidebending.
What motions are observed at the atlanto-axial (AA) joint?	Primarily rotation. A minor amount of flexion/extension is present.

DIAGNOSIS

What primary observations should be made when examining the neck?	1. Erythema (blanching) 2. Skin temperature 3. Skin texture 4. Skin moisture or dryness 5. Lymph nodes 6. Muscle spasm 7. Thyroid gland 8. Scars 9. Lordosis (increased/decreased) 10. Tracheal position 11. Jugular venous distention 12. Carotid bruits 13. Neck motion
How is sidebending of the cervical spine assessed?	Translating the vertebra (or occiput) to one side will test sidebending to the opposite side. For example, translating C_3 to the left by pushing it medially from the right will test right sidebending of C_3 on C_4.
How is rotation of the cervical spine assessed?	Firm contact is made with the articular pillars of the cervical vertebra on the posterior aspect of the neck. Pushing one articular pillar anterior will test rotation to the opposite side. For example, pushing the left articular pillar of C_4 anterior will test right rotation of C_4 on C_5. Also, static palpation of the articular pillars and assessing for symmetry can also give an idea of rotation of the cervical vertebrae—the vertebra is rotated to the side of the posterior articular pillar.
How is motion at the AA joint tested?	The neck is gently flexed to its barrier. The head is then rotated to either side and checked for its freedom and barrier to rotation.
What is the correct method of palpating the thyroid gland?	Ask patient to slightly extend head. Using two hands, examiner palpates anterior neck below thyroid cartilage (at level of C_5 to C_7). Having the patient swallow may assist in bringing the thyroid anterior and superior for palpation.

SPECIAL TESTS

How is the Spurling maneuver performed?	Patient may be supine or seated. Examiner applies a compressive force from the top of the patient's head through the patient's cervical spine. Adding sidebending to the side of the patient's neurologic symptoms may increase specificity of the test.
What is a positive Spurling maneuver?	Reproduction or increase in the patient's neurologic or radicular symptoms in the upper extremity indicates a positive test result.
How does the Spurling maneuver test the cervical nerve roots?	Compression of the cervical spine causes narrowing of the intervertebral foramina. Any preexisting narrowing of the foramina is thus exaggerated leading to reproduction or increase in the patient's symptoms.
What is the distraction test (A.K.A. reverse Spurling maneuver)?	With the patient supine, the examiner cups the base of the patient's head and distracts the cervical vertebrae. This in turn relieves any narrowing of the cervical intervertebral foramina.
What is indicative of a positive distraction test result?	Temporary decrease or relief of the patient's neurologic or radicular symptoms with distraction is a positive sign.

TREATMENT

What are the direct effects of treatment of cervical vertebral somatic dysfunctions?	↑ neck range of motion, ↓ muscle spasms, ↓ fascial strains, ↓ ligamentous tension, improved motion of ribs 1 and 2, and improved respiratory diaphragm function (via phrenic n.).
What different treatment modalities are used in treatment of the vertebrae?	Counterstrain, facilitated positional release, muscle energy, high velocity low amplitude (HVLA), balanced ligamentous tension, myofascial, Chapman's reflex, trigger points.
When performing HVLA of the cervical spine, what direction is the thrust directed?	**Most commonly, a rotational thrust is used during HVLA of the cervical spine. Due to the varied planes of the cervical facets, the rotational thrust should be directed as follows:** • **C_2 and C_3: Toward contralateral eye** • **C_4 and C_5: Straight across in the horizontal plane** • **C_6 and C_7: Toward contralateral axilla.**

What are the specific contraindications to HVLA of the cervical spine?

Other than the general contraindications outlined in Chapter 1, those specific to the cervical vertebrae when using HVLA include rheumatoid arthritis, compromised arterial supply to the head (vertebral and carotid aa.), acute whiplash, and spondylolysis.

What is the general rule for counterstrain of the cervical region?

The anterior cervical tenderpoints require flexion (except C_4) and the posterior cervical tenderpoints require extension (except C_3) (Figure 3.16A and Figure 3.16B).

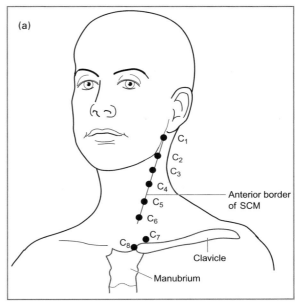

FIGURE 3.16A – Anterior cervical tenderpoints.

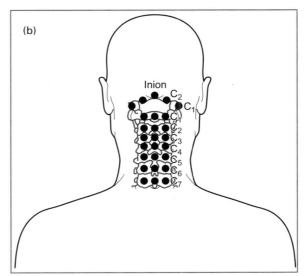

FIGURE 3.16B – Posterior cervical tenderpoints.

How is the anterior tenderpoint for C$_4$ treated?	Patient is supine with the head hanging off the table supported by the physician's hands. The patient's neck is extended, sidebent away and rotated away up to the level of C$_4$.
What is the treatment for the posterior tenderpoint at C$_3$?	Patient is supine. Physician flexes patient's neck to the level of C$_3$. If necessary, the physician may add sidebending toward and rotation away from the tenderpoint.

4 THORACIC

GROSS ANATOMY OVERVIEW

Dermatomes from the Thoracic Spine (Figure 4.1)

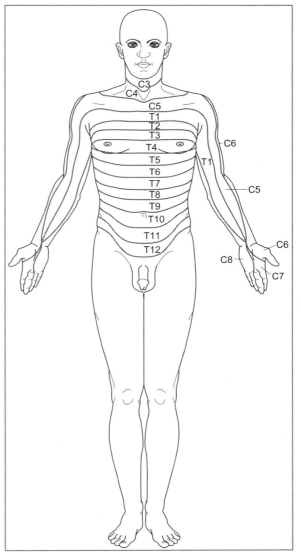

FIGURE 4.1 – Dermatomes from the thoracic spine.

Identify the following structures (Figure 4.2):

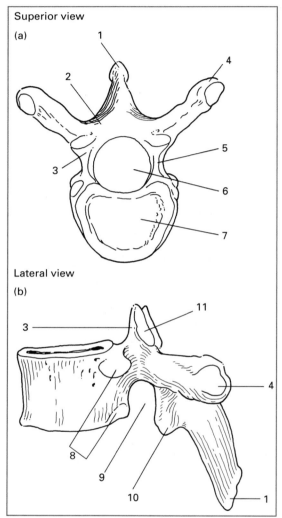

Superior view
(a)

Lateral view
(b)

FIGURE 4.2 – Typical thoracic vertebrae.

1. Spinous process (SP)
2. Lamina
3. Superior articular process
4. Transverse process (TP)
5. Pedicle
6. Vertebral foramen
7. Vertebral body
8. Demifacets (for rib heads)
9. Intervertebral foramen
10. Inferior articular process
11. Superior articular facet.

What is the primary curvature of the thoracic spine?   Kyphosis.

List three features of the thoracic vertebrae that distinguish them from the cervical and lumbar vertebrae.

1. Costal facets (demifacets) on their bodies
2. Costal facets on their transverse processes
3. Long spinous processes.

Which vertebrae have upper and lower demifacets for the ribheads?

The typical vertebrae T_2–T_9.

How do the costal facets vary among thoracic vertebrae?

T_1: single facet for the head of the first rib and a demifacet for the top of the second rib.

T_{10}: only one costal facet located on the body and pedicle.

T_{11} and T_{12}: only one costal facet located on their pedicles.

 Memory Aid: All of these vertebrae with varying costal facets have "**1**" in their number.

How do the levels of the TPs relate to the level of the SPs in thoracic vertebrae?

Rule 1: T_1–T_3, SPs at the same level as their TPs

Rule 2: T_4–T_6, SPs located half the distance between their TP and the next (lower) TP

Rule 3: T_7–T_9, SPs at the level of the next (lower) TP

T10: Follows Rule 3

T11: Follows Rule 2

T12: Follows Rule 1

 Memory Aid: Rule of 3s

What landmarks may be used when palpating thoracic vertebrae?

T_1: below vertebral prominens (C_7) and it articulates with the first rib.

T_2: manubrium/sternal notch (anterior).

T_3: SP is at the level of the spine of scapula.

T_7: Rib 7 is found at the level of the inferior angle of scapula and can be followed medially to find T_7. Xiphoid process is at the level of T_7.

T_{12}: Rib 12 (last rib) articulates with T_{12}.

Identify the following structures (Figure 4.3):

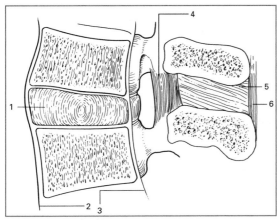

FIGURE 4.3 – Vertebral ligaments.

1. Intervertebral disc (IV disc)
2. Anterior longitudinal ligament
3. Posterior longitudinal ligament
4. Ligamentum flavum
5. Interspinous ligament
6. Supraspinous ligament.

What is the anterior longitudinal ligament?	Strong fibrous band connecting the anterolateral surfaces of the vertebral bodies and IV discs. It helps maintain stability and prevents hyperextension (see Figure 4.3).
What is the posterior longitudinal ligament?	A thin fibrous band that runs along the posterior aspect of the vertebral bodies within the vertebral canal. Its helps prevent hyperflexion and posterior disc herniation (see Figure 4.3).
What ligament joins the laminae of adjacent vertebral arches?	Ligamenta flava (see Figure 4.3).
How is the interspinous ligament different from the supraspinous ligament?	The interspinous ligament is a thinner ligament that joins the root of one SP to the apex of the SP below. The supraspinous ligament is a broader ligament connecting the apices of multiple adjacent SPs (see Figure 4.3).
What is the major determinant of the range of motion between vertebrae?	The size of the IV disc relative to the vertebral bodies. The thoracic spine has the smallest IV disc to vertebral body ratio. 🐛 **Memory Aid:** Decrease in ROM = decrease in ratio
What parts of a rib articulate with vertebrae?	The head of the rib (with the vertebral body) and tubercle (with the TP). *(See Figure 5.2 in Chapter 5: Ribs.)*
Why are the bodies of T_5–T_8 flattened on their left side?	Due to the pressure from the descending aorta.
What is the major blood supply of thoracic vertebrae?	Posterior intercostal arteries.
What is the nervous innervation to the deep (A.K.A. intrinsic) muscles of the back?	Dorsal rami of spinal nerves.
What muscles constitute the following layers of the deep back muscles:	
Superficial layer	Splenii mm.
Intermediate layer	Erector spinae mm. • Iliocostalii mm. • Longissimus mm. • Spinalii mm.

Deep layer

Transversospinal mm.

- Semispinalii mm.
- Multifidi mm.
- Rotatores mm.

Interspinales mm.
Intertransversarii mm.
Levatores costarum mm.

CLINICAL ANATOMY

Where is local anesthetic injected when performing an intercostal nerve block?	It is injected in the paravertebral line (a vertical line connecting the tips of transverse processes).
Does intercostal nerve block create complete loss of sensation in the specific dermatome affected?	No, any particular area of skin typically receives sensory innervation from two or more adjacent nerves. Thus, there is considerable overlapping of dermatomes and their respective sensory innervation.
What is scoliosis?	A lateral curvature of the spine greater than 10 degrees.
List the major causes of scoliosis.	• Congenital • Infantile • Paralytic • Neurofibromatosis • Idiopathic or adolescent
What are the anomalies associated with congenital scoliosis?	Hemi-vertebrae, fused vertebrae, congenital paralysis, spina bifida, and cerebral palsy.
What is the most common age, gender, and side that patients with infantile scoliosis present?	Boys younger than 3 years old without vertebral anomalies. It is more common on the left and approximately 90% of cases resolve spontaneously.
What type of vertebrae is most commonly affected in idiopathic scoliosis?	Thoracic.
What is the most common age, gender, and side that patients with idiopathic scoliosis present?	10-year-old girls with curves that are convex to the right. There may also be compensatory curves above and below the primary curve.
What is non-structural (A.K.A. functional) scoliosis?	A spinal curvature that corrects on lying down or when the underlying cause is removed. For example, the curve may be the result of a short leg, hip deformity, muscle spasm, prolapsed disc, tumor, or spinal infection.

How can the degree of scoliosis be measured?

The Cobb method involves measuring angles that appear on plain film radiographs.

Mild scoliosis: 5 to 15 degrees.
Moderate scoliosis: 20 to 45 degrees.
Severe scoliosis: > 50 degrees.

Describe the measurement of an angle in the Cobb method.

One line is drawn parallel to the first affected vertebra at the top of the curve and another line through the bottom of the lowest affected vertebra. The angle of the intersection of two lines drawn perpendicular to the above two lines indicates the Cobb angle (Figure 4.4).

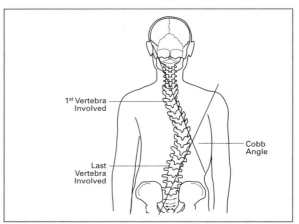

FIGURE 4.4 – Cobb angle.

What is Pott's disease?	Tuberculosis infection of the spine.
How are the thoracic vertebrae affected by an aneurysm of the thoracic aorta?	The bodies of T_5–T_8 can become partially eroded from the pressure of the aneurysm.
What is the classic distribution pattern for herpes zoster infections (A.K.A. shingles)?	Herpes zoster is a viral infection of the spinal ganglia. Thus, when the infection is active, its clinical presentation is localized to the area of dermatomal and myotomal distribution of the spinal ganglia. Typically, red painful vesicular lesions will appear in the affected dermatome.

OSTEOPATHIC PRINCIPLES

What are the three planes of motion for the thoracic spine?	1. Flexion/extension in the sagittal plane. 2. Sidebending (lateral flexion) in the coronal plane. 3. Rotation in the transverse (horizontal) plane.
What is the primary motion exhibited in thoracic spine?	Rotation. Then, lateral flexion > flexion > extension.
Which part of the vertebral column exhibits the most limited range of motion (ROM)? Why?	Thoracic spine due to: • Presence of thoracic cage (ribs and sternum) • Least "IV disc:vertebral body" ratio
What laws best describe the coupled motions of the thoracic spine?	Fryette's Principles.
What law is used to describe group dysfunctions?	Fryette's Principle I.
What law is used to describe single vertebral dysfunctions?	Fryette's Principle II.
What is a rib hump?	A unilateral posterior protrusion of a group of ribs upon flexion of the vertebral column (on the same side as the convexity of the curve). This clinical finding is indicative of scoliosis.

What organs/regions do the following pre-ganglionic sympathetic nerves innervate?

T1–T4	**Head and neck**
T1–T6	**Heart and lungs**
T1–T8	**Upper extremity**
T2–T8	**Esophagus**
T5–T9	**Upper GI tract (up to the second part of the duodenum)**
T10–T11	**Midgut (from third part of the duodenum to the second third of the transverse colon)**
	Adrenal glands
	Kidneys
	Upper ureter
T10–L2	**Prostate and prostatic urethra (in males)**
	Uterus and cervix (in females)
T11–L2	**Lower extremity**
T12	**Appendix**
T12–L1	**Lower ureter**
T12–L2	**Hindgut (up to the pectinate line)**
	Bladder

DIAGNOSIS

What primary observations should be made when examining the thoracic spine?	1. Erythema (blanching) 2. Skin temperature 3. Skin texture 4. Skin moisture or dryness 5. Muscle spasm 6. Scars 7. Rib humps 8. Kyphosis (increased/decreased)
What is a quick and effective method of evaluating a possible traumatic vertebral fracture?	Placing a small amount of pressure on each individual SP to elicit any pain response.
What are the different types of somatic dysfunctions found in the thoracic vertebrae?	1. Type I (group dysfunction) 2. Type II (single vertebra dysfunction)

Define type I dysfunctions.	A type I somatic dysfunction consists of three or more consecutive vertebrae that follow Fryette's Law I (with rotation and sidebending in opposite directions in a neutral spine).
Define type II dysfunctions.	A type II somatic dysfunction consists of a single vertebra that follows Fryette's Law II (with rotation and sidebending in same directions in a non-neutral spine).
Name the type of dysfunction exhibited by a patient with four consecutive vertebrae rotated and side-bent in the same direction.	This is still a type II dysfunction because the patient has four consecutive single vertebra dysfunctions (rotation and sidebending in the same direction). Upon further motion testing of these four vertebrae, each segment must be found in a position of either flexion or extension.

Define the type and name of the following somatic dysfunctions:

Upon motion testing, T_1 is flexed, rotated right, and sidebent to the right.	Type II somatic dysfunction. T_1 F R_R S_R
T_2–T_5 are neutral in extension and flexion, but rotated to the right and sidebent to the left.	Type I somatic dysfunction. T_2–T_5 N R_R S_L
A status post-myocardial infarction (MI) patient is found to have a second thoracic vertebra that freely rotates and sidebends to the left. Motion becomes more symmetric with extension.	Type II somatic dysfunction. T_2 E R_L S_L
A patient with known history of gastro-esophageal reflux disease presents with mid-back pain. Structural findings include: • T_5 F R_R S_R • T_6 F R_R S_R • T_7 F R_R S_R • T_8 F R_R S_R • T_9 E R_R S_R	The patient has five individual type II somatic dysfunctions. This is not a group curve because each vertebra has a flexion or extension component to them. In each case, sidebending and rotation are on the same side.
A teenager comes to a clinic with mild respiratory discomfort. Upon palpation, a curve with concavity to the right is noted from T_4–T_8. Another curve with convexity to the right is noted from T_{10}–L_1.	The patient has an "S" type curve made of two type I group curves. T_4–T_8 N R_L S_R T_{10}–L_1 N R_R S_L In this case, T_9 is called the "transitional vertebra."

43

SPECIAL TESTS

Describe the screening test for scoliosis.	**Adam's test: Patient stands with feet shoulder width apart and is asked to slowly bend forward. Examiner checks for posterior protrusion of ribs (rib hump).**
During a well-child visit, a 5-year-old girl is noted to have a group curve at T_5–T_8 N R_R S_L. Where can a rib hump be found?	A rib hump may be found on the right side (ribs 5–8) because the rotation of the vertebrae of the group curve causes the TPs to protrude posteriorly. This posterior position of the TPs results in posterior protrusion of respective ribs on that same side (rib hump).

TREATMENT

What are the direct effects of treatment of thoracic spine somatic dysfunctions?	↑ thoracic ROM, normalize sympathetic outflow, ↓ muscle spasms, ↓ fascial strains, ↓ ligamentous tension, and improved rib motion.
How does treatment of the thoracic spine affect the sympathetic outflow from the thoracic region?	The sympathetic innervation to the body is delivered through spinal nerves T1 to L2 (or L3). Moreover, the sympathetic trunk and ganglia lie lateral to the vertebral bodies near the pedicles. Treatment of vertebral facilitations in the thoracic region can thus normalize sympathetic nervous outflow.
What vertebra should be targeted in treatment of a "C"-shaped (single-sided) scoliotic curve?	The vertebra(e) in the middle of the curve.
What are the specific contraindications to high velocity low amplitude (HVLA) of the thoracic vertebra?	Aside from the general contraindications mentioned in Chapter 1, those specific to the thoracic vertebrae when using HVLA include MI, acute asthma exacerbation, shortness of breath, dyspnea, pleuritic chest pain, aortic aneurysm, open thoracic cavity wound/trauma, pneumothorax/hemothorax.

Anterior and Posterior Thoracic Tenderpoints
(Figure 4.5A and Figure 4.5B)

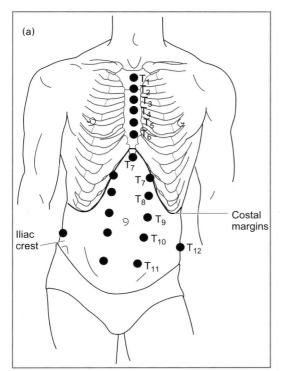

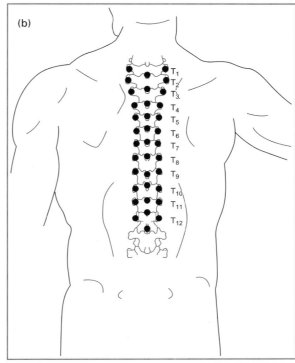

FIGURE 4.5 – A: Anterior thoracic tenderpoints. B: Posterior thoracic tenderpoints.

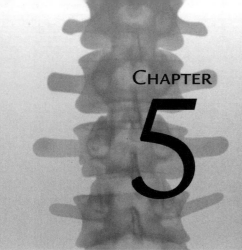

5 RIBS

GROSS ANATOMY OVERVIEW

Rib Cage (Figure 5.1)

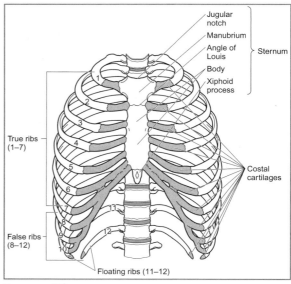

FIGURE 5.1 – Rib cage.

Where on the sternum does the second rib insert?

Angle of Louis (A.K.A. sternal angle).

Which ribs are considered atypical?

Ribs 1, 2, 10, 11, and 12 are atypical.

 Memory Aid: All the atypical ribs have either a "**one**" or "**two**" in their number (**1**, **2**, **10**, **11**, and **12**)

What parts of a rib articulate with vertebrae?

The head and tubercle (Figure 5.2).

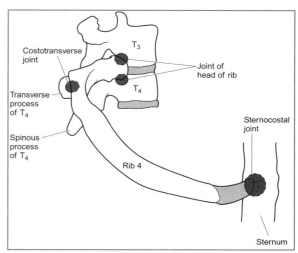

FIGURE 5.2 – Rib articulations.

Where do the heads of the typical ribs articulate with the vertebrae?

At the superior and inferior costal facets (except for the atypical ribs) forming the joint of head of rib.

Where does the tubercle of the rib articulate with the vertebrae?

At the transverse costal facet forming the costotransverse articulation.

The joint of head of rib and the costotransverse articulation form what joint?

Costovertebral joint.

Rib Osteology (Figure 5.3)

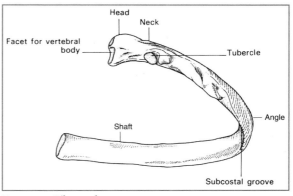

FIGURE 5.3 – Rib osteology.

What muscles attach to the first rib?

Middle and **A**nterior scalene muscles (from the neck) along with **S**ubclavius and **S**erratus anterior muscles (from anterior chest wall).

 Memory Aid: A **MASS** of muscles attach to the 1st rib.

What vessels form a groove on the first rib?	Subclavian a. and subclavian v. form the two subclavian grooves separated by the scalene tubercle.
What muscles attach to the second rib?	Posterior scalene muscle (from the neck) along with serratus anterior muscle (from anterior chest wall).
What muscle(s) attach to ribs 3–5?	The pectoralis minor muscle attaches near their costal cartilages.
What muscles attach to the 12th rib?	Posterior origin of the diaphragm (through the lateral arcuate ligament), and quadratus lumborum.

Identify the following intercostal structures (Figure 5.4):

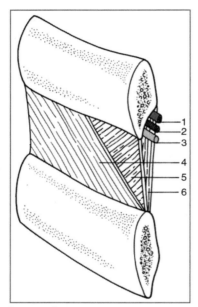

FIGURE 5.4 – Intercostal space.

1. Intercostal vein
2. Intercostal artery
3. Intercostal nerve
4. External intercostal m.
5. Internal intercostal m.
6. Innermost intercostal m.

In what directions do the fibers of the intercostal muscles run?

External intercostal mm.: inferoanteriorly.

 Memory Aid: External intercostal fibers run in the same direction as your hands in your pockets.

Internal intercostal mm.: inferoposteriorly (right angle to external intercostal mm.)

Innermost intercostal mm.: inferoposteriorly (same direction as internal intercostal mm.)

What anterior abdominal wall muscles are continuous with the thoracic cage muscles?

External intercostal mm.: External abdominal oblique mm.

Internal intercostal mm.: Internal abdominal oblique mm.

Transversus thoracis mm.: Transversus abdominis mm.

What are the serratus anterior muscles?

They overlie the lateral surface of the thorax. Their action includes protracting the scapula and rotating the scapula to the glenoid-up position. May also serve as an accessory muscle of respiration.

 Memory Aid: Serratus (in Latin) means toothed like a saw. This is how the anterior and posterior edges of all serratus muscles appear.

What structures pass between the internal intercostal mm. and the innermost intercostal mm.?

Posterior intercostal <u>v</u>ein, posterior intercostal <u>a</u>rtery, and intercostal <u>n</u>erve (see Figure 5.4).

 Memory Aid: <u>VAN</u> stands for the Intercostal <u>V</u>ein, <u>A</u>rtery, <u>N</u>erve.

Are the neurovascular structures located superiorly or inferiorly within their respective intercostal space?

Superiorly.

 Memory Aid: A VAN is taller (more superior) than most cars.

Identify the branches of the subclavian a.
(Figure 5.5):

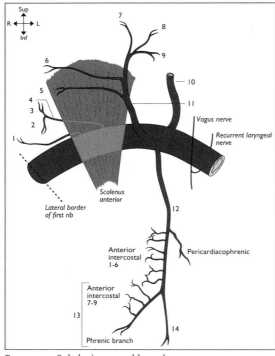

1. Dorsal scapular a.
2. Superior intercostal a.
3. Deep cervical a.
4. Costocervical trunk
5. Suprascapular a.
6. Superficial cervical a.
7. Ascending cervical a.
8. Inferior laryngeal a.
9. Inferior thyroid a.
10. Vertebral a.
11. Thyrocervical trunk
12. Internal thoracic (mammary) a.
13. Musculophrenic a.
14. Superior epigastric a.

FIGURE 5.5 – Subclavian a. and branches.

Thoracic Cage Venous Drainage (Figure 5.6)

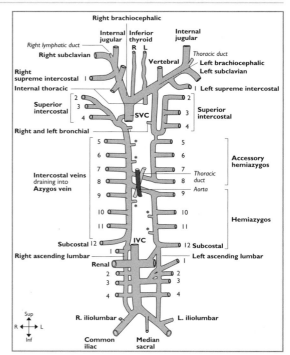

FIGURE 5.6 – Thoracic cage venous drainage.

Describe the relation of the intercostal nerves to spinal nerves.

The ventral rami of spinal nn. T1–T11 form the intercostal nerves that run within the intercostal spaces. The ventral ramus of the T12 spinal n. runs inferior to the 12th rib and is called the subcostal nerve.

What is the relation of the ribs to the sympathetic ganglia/trunk (paravertebral ganglia chain)?

The trunk/ganglia lie anterior to the head of each rib (Figure 5.7).

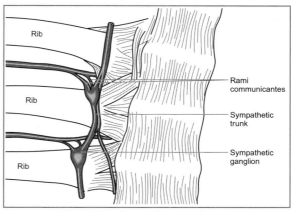

FIGURE 5.7 – Relationship of sympathetic trunk.

List the bony borders of the thoracic inlet.

First rib, clavicle, manubrium, and T$_1$.

 ***Memory Aid:* The 1st of each type of bone:**

- **1st rib**
- **1st part of sternum (manubrium)**
- **1st thoracic vertebra**
- **1st bone of the upper extremity (clavicle) (Figure 5.8).**

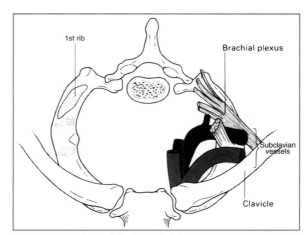

FIGURE 5.8 – Borders of the thoracic inlet.

What soft-tissue structures form the diaphragm of the thoracic inlet?

Scalenes (**P**osterior, **A**nterior, and **M**iddle), **S**CM, **I**nvesting layer of deep cervical fascia, **P**arietal pleura, and **S**ibson's fascia (suprapleural membrane).

 Memory Aid: **PAM SIPS** her drink.

What structures pass through the thoracic inlet?

Common carotid aa., subclavian aa. and vv., external and internal jugular vv., thoracic duct, brachial plexus, phrenic nerves, vagus nerves, trachea, and esophagus (Figure 5.9).

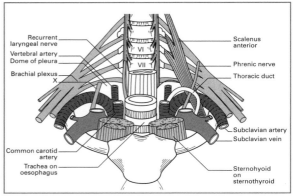

FIGURE 5.9 – Contents of the thoracic inlet.

CLINICAL ANATOMY

What structures will most likely be injured with fracture of the first rib?

Brachial plexus and subclavian vessels. (*Hint: Think of structures in the thoracic inlet.*)

What is a flail chest (A.K.A. stove-in chest)?

Multiple rib fractures resulting in paradoxical movement of the thorax with respiration (outward with expiration and inward with inspiration). This results in severe pain with poor ventilation.

How do people with cervical ribs present?

Most are asymptomatic but can be found on palpation. Symptoms may result from compression of the inferior trunk of the brachial plexus and subclavian vessels, resulting in pain in the fourth and fifth digits and ischemic muscle pain.

What is most common site of sternal fracture?

Sternal angle (A.K.A. angle of Louis)

What is the ideal location to place a chest tube (tube thoracostomy) and why?

Thoracocentesis is often used to treat pneumothorax or drain pleural fluid. A thoracostomy tube should be placed at the fourth intercostal space just above the fifth rib (to avoid injury to the intercostal neurovascular bundle located directly under each rib).

OSTEOPATHIC PRINCIPLES

Where is the axis for rib motion?

The axis of motion for ribs passes through the costotransverse articulation and the joint of head of rib (Figure 5.10).

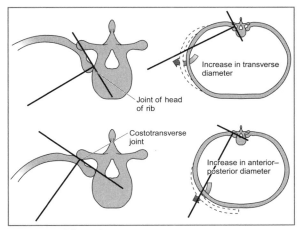

FIGURE 5.10 – Rib motion axes.

Name and describe the different types of motion for ribs 1–10.

Pump handle: Motion of the ribs where the anterior end elevates with a fixed posterior end to increase the anteroposterior diameter of the rib cage (Figure 5.11A).

Bucket handle: Motion of the ribs where the lateral portion elevates with fixed anterior and posterior ends resulting in an increased transverse diameter of the rib cage (Figure 5.11B).

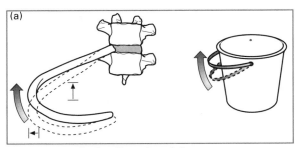

FIGURE 5.11A – Bucket handle motion of ribs.

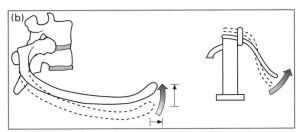

FIGURE 5.11B – Pump handle motion of ribs.

Which ribs exhibit pump handle motion?	Primarily upper ribs 1 through 3. However, ribs 4 through 10 also exhibit some pump handle motion.
Which ribs exhibit bucket handle motion?	Primarily lower ribs 8 through 10. However, ribs one through seven also exhibit some bucket handle motion.
What type of motion do the 11th and 12th ribs exhibit?	Caliper motions: Lateral ends move postero-infero-laterally by action of quadratus lumborum m. contraction during inspiration. Theoretically, this should increase anteroposterior and transverse diameters and stabilize the origins of the diaphragm (Figure 5.12).

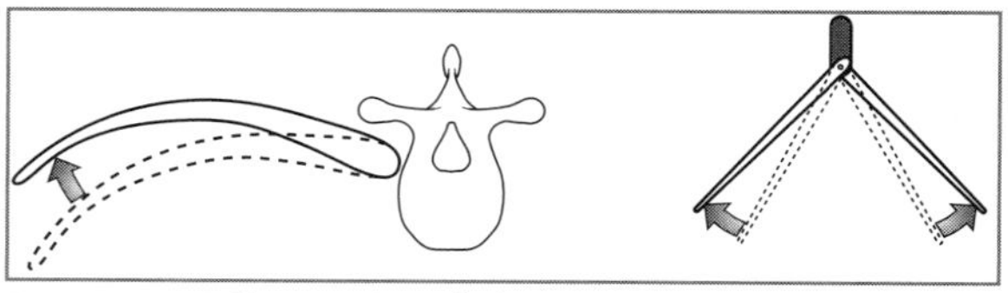

FIGURE 5.12 – Caliper motion of ribs 11 and 12.

List nine structures affected by the ribs.	1. Lymphatics system 2. Venous circulation 3. Sympathetic nervous system 4. Abdominal diaphragm 5. Thoracic inlet 6. Lungs 7. Heart 8. Local soft tissue (muscles, ligaments, fascia, etc.) 9. Other ribs and vertebrae.
How does the motion of the ribs affect lymphatic and venous flow through the body?	The negative and positive intra-thoracic pressures (created by rib motion during respiration) form the primary driving force for lymphatic and venous return.
What is the effect of the ribs on the thoracic inlet?	The first rib forms one of the borders of the thoracic inlet and therefore can affect all structures forming the diaphragm and passing through the thoracic inlet (listed above).
How do ribs affect the lungs?	Sympathetic innervations, lymphatic drainage and lung expansion are all affected by the position and motion of the ribs.

How do the ribs relate to heart function?	Sympathetic innervations, venous return, heart expansion, and the central tendon of diaphragm are all factors that can be affected by the ribs to change heart function.
What is the effect of the ribs on the heart during inspiration?	By expanding the thoracic cavity, heart expansion is improved and venous return is increased (allowing better atrial filling). Inspiration also prolongs ejection of blood from right ventricle, but shortens ejection from the left ventricle leading to a split S_2 sound during inspiration.
How can one rib affect surrounding ribs?	**When a rib is restricted in its normal motion, it may cause its surrounding ribs to exhibit the same dysfunction. For example, 1) if a rib is unable to move inferiorly, it may prevent the ribs above it from moving inferiorly; and 2) if a rib is unable to move superiorly, it may prevent the ribs below it from moving superiorly.**

DIAGNOSIS

What are general signs and symptoms associated with rib dysfunction?	Shortness of breath (SOB), dyspnea, pain with respiration, chest tightness, tenderness, coughing/sneezing, cyanosis, pallor, edema, intercostal retractions, prominent subcostal margins, uneven shoulders, and ↓ neck and shoulder range of motion.
How can one identify a fractured rib on physical exam?	**Anteroposterior compression of the chest will help distinguish a fracture from a soft tissue injury. Increased local pain suggests rib fracture.**
Describe the following rib somatic dysfunctions:	
Inhalation dysfunction	The rib is in an inspiratory position. It is free to move into further inspiration, however is restricted during expiration. (A.K.A. exhalation restriction)
Exhalation dysfunction	The rib is in an expiratory position. The rib may freely move further in expiration, but is restricted during inspiration. (A.K.A. inhalation restriction)
Elevated rib	The rib is superior relative to its normal position. Elevated ribs generally correlate with inhalation dysfunctions.
Depressed rib	The rib is inferior relative to its normal position. Depressed ribs generally correlate with exhalation dysfunctions.

Anterior rib	The rib is anterior relative to its normal position. Rib can be palpated with greater anterior protrusion.
Posterior rib	The rib is posterior relative to its normal position. Rib can be palpated with greater posterior protrusion.

What is a group rib somatic dysfunction?	When two or more consecutive ribs exhibit the same dysfunction.

Where can one evaluate function for:

Bucket handle motion for ribs 1–10?	Place hands flat over anterior surface of ribs allowing fingers to span laterally.
Pump handle motion for ribs 1–10?	Place medial side of hands on either side of sternum and medial edge of costal cartilage.
Rib 1?	Palpate rib 1 at three locations: 1) posterior aspect near TP of T_1; 2) supero-medial aspect of anterior half (postero-superior to medial end of clavicle); and 3) inferior to medial end of clavicle.
Individual rib (ribs 2–10)?	Approach the rib laterally with both hands. The tips of your thumbs should meet at the mid-axillary line with index fingers spanning the rib medially on either side.
Individual rib (ribs 11 or 12)?	Place thumb over head of rib and allow index finger to span the posterior aspect of the rib laterally.
Abdominal diaphragm	Tuck fingers under costal margins with fingertips pointing superiorly.

Describe the following deformities of the thoracic cage:	Increased antero-posterior diameter. Often the result of chronic obstructive pulmonary disease (see Figure 5.13A).
Barrel chest	

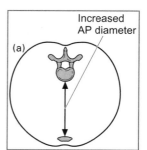

FIGURE 5.13 – Deformities of the thoracic cage. A: barrel.

Pectus carinatum (pigeon chest)

Increased antero-posterior diameter with anterior sternum and depressed costal cartilages (see Figure 5.13B).

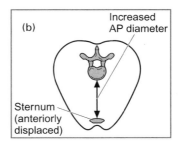

FIGURE 5.13 – B: pigeon.

Pectus excavatum (funnel chest)

Depression of the lower sternum that can compress the heart and great vessels (see Figure 5.13C).

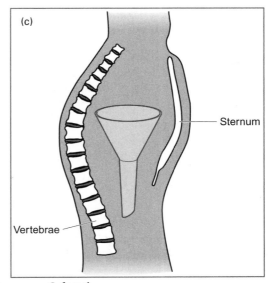

FIGURE 5.13 – C: funnel.

What is a rib hump?

When a patient bends forward, certain ribs may protrude posteriorly. Generally, this test is used to screen for scoliosis.

(See Chapter 4: Thoracic—Special Tests)

TREATMENT

What are the direct effects of treatment of thoracic cage somatic dysfunction?	Improved rib motion, ↓ muscle spasms, ↓ fascial strains, ↓ ligamentous tension, ↑ abdominal diaphragm excursion, and ↑ thoracic cavity expansion.
How does treatment of the rib affect the sympathetic outflow from the thoracic region?	**Due to the proximity of the sympathetic ganglia/ trunk to the heads of the ribs, treatment of the ribs can decrease facilitation around the sympathetic ganglia/trunk. This results in normalization of sympathetic outflow from the thoracic region.**
How does OMT to the ribs and associated soft tissue improve respiratory function?	By improving the motion of the ribs, the expansion of intra-thoracic volume improves, ↓ use of accessory muscles of respiration, allowing better lung expansion/filling and more efficient respiratory function with less energy expenditure.
How does treatment of the ribs affect lymphatic and venous return?	Treatment of the ribs improves thoracic cavity and abdominal diaphragm excursion. This enhances the negative and positive intra-thoracic pressures formed during respiration. It is these pressures that form the primary drive for lymphatic and venous return from the entire body, hence, resulting in ↓ edema, improved lymphatic/immune function, and better circulation.
What are the cardiovascular effects of treatment of the thoracic cage?	↑ venous return, ↑ thoracic cavity expansion and normalized sympathetic innervations results in ↑ coronary oxygenation/perfusion, ↑ cardiac expansion, ↑ atrial/ventricular filling, ↑ cardiac output, and ↑ cardiac contractility.
Which rib should be the primary target in treatment in group inhalation dysfunctions?	**The most inferior rib in this group dysfunction must be treated because the inhaled position of the rib will keep the ribs immediately above it in a position of inhalation.**
Which rib should be the primary target in treatment in group exhalation dysfunctions?	**The most superior rib in this group dysfunction must be treated because the exhaled position of the rib will keep the ribs immediately below it in a position of exhalation.**
What different treatment modalities may be used in the treatment of the ribs?	Rib raising, counterstrain (CS), faciliated positional release, muscle energy, high velocity low amplitude (HVLA), balanced ligamentous tension, ligamentous articular strain, myofascial, Chapman's reflex, trigger points.

How is rib raising performed?	By applying pressure to the heads of the ribs and moving them anterolaterally.
How does rib raising affect the autonomic nervous system?	Due to the proximity of the sympathetic ganglion chain to the head of the ribs, rib raising can be used to normalize sympathetic outflow from the thoracic region.
Where are the CS tenderpoints located anteriorly?	Generally, the anterior tenderpoints are located at two locations, the costosternal joint and anterior-axillary line on the respective ribs. Anterior rib tenderpoints are generally associated with depressed ribs (Figure 5.14A).

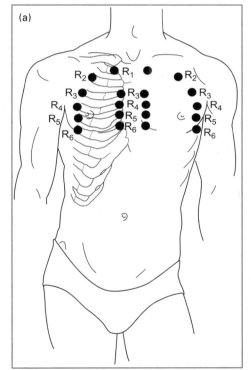

FIGURE 5.14A – Anterior rib tenderpoints.

Where are the posterior CS tenderpoints located?

The posterior rib tenderpoints are located at the respective rib angles. They are generally associated with elevated ribs (Figure 5.14B).

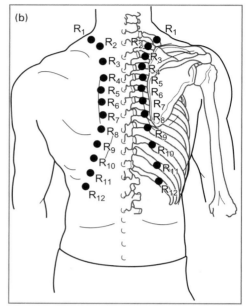

FIGURE 5.14B – Posterior rib tenderpoints.

How long do you hold the CS tenderpoints at their mobile point?

120 seconds (not 90 seconds like other areas of the body!)

What are contraindications to rib raising?

Fracture of the thoracic spine and/or the rib being treated.

What are the specific contraindications to HVLA of the ribs?

Aside from the general contraindications mentioned in Chapter 1, those specific to the ribs when using HVLA include myocardial infarction, acute asthma exacerbation, SOB, dyspnea, pleuritic chest pain, and aortic aneurysm.

When dysfunctions are found at a rib and its corresponding vertebra, which dysfunction should be treated first?

There is no universal answer. Treatment should be based on individual findings. The examiner should distinguish between the primary (key) lesion and its resulting (secondary) compensation and treat accordingly.

CHAPTER

6 LUMBAR

GROSS ANATOMY OVERVIEW

Dermatomes from the Lumbar Spine (Figure 6.1)

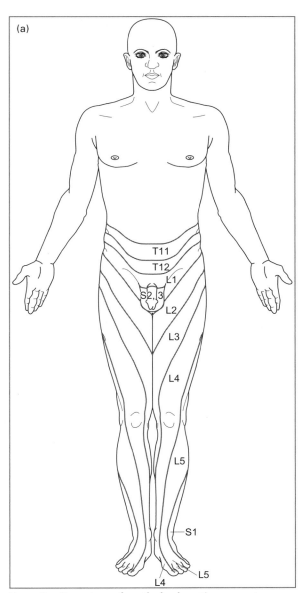

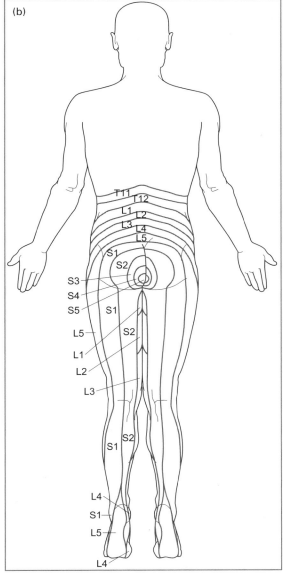

FIGURE 6.1 – Dermatomes from the lumbar spine.

What is the normal curvature of the lumbar spine?

Lordosis (considered a secondary curvature because it develops after the fetal period).

 Memory Aid: <u>L</u>umbar → <u>L</u>ordotic

Name the largest movable vertebrae in the entire spine.

L_5 (also carries the largest amount of weight).

What structure (unique to lumbar vertebrae) is located on the posterior surface of their superior articular processes?

Mamillary processes (attachment for multifidus and intertransversarii mm.) (Figure 6.2).

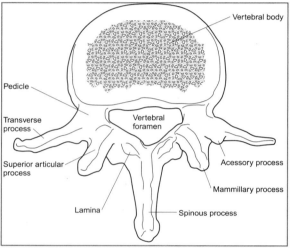

FIGURE 6.2 – Lumbar vertebrae.

What two structures make up an intervertebral disc?

Annulus fibrosis (circumferential) and nucleus pulposus (central).

Which intervertebral disc structure is nearly 90% water?

Nucleus pulposus (giving this structure enough turgor to fit tightly between vertebrae and within the annulus fibrosis).

In adults, what vertebral level usually marks the end of the spinal cord? In embryos? At birth?

The spinal cord extends to L_2 in adults, occupies the full length of the vertebral canal in embryos, and extends to L_2/L_3 at birth (Figure 6.3).

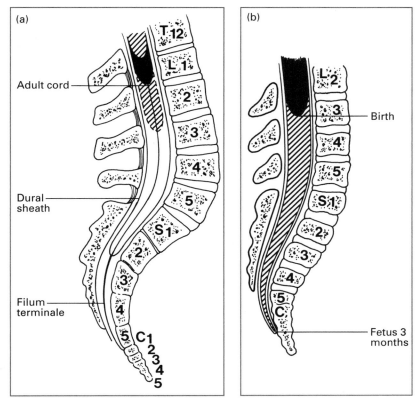

FIGURE 6.3 – A: Spinal cord in adults. B: Spinal cord at birth and in 3-month-old fetus.

CLINICAL ANATOMY

Describe spina bifida.

A congenital anomaly where the laminae of L_5 and/or S_1 fail to fuse normally. Patient presentation can vary from asymptomatic to severe neurologic deficits depending on the type of spina bifida.

What are two types of spina bifida?

1. Spina bifida occulta: defect is concealed by skin and tuft of hair, minor vertebral anomaly with no symptomatology.
2. Spina bifida cystica: complete lack of fusion of arches with herniation of spinal cord structures and neurologic symptoms.

What spinal cord structures commonly herniate in spina bifida cystica?

1. **Meninges (meningocele)**
2. **Spinal cord and meninges (meningomyelocele)**
3. **Failure of fusion of neural tube with ependymal layer exposure—rachischisis (myelocele) (Figure 6.4).**

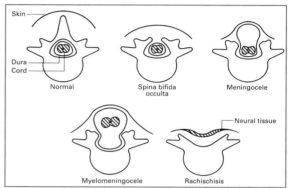

FIGURE 6.4 – Types of spina bifida.

List common symptoms associated with a meningomyelocele.

Lower limb paralysis, lack of motor and/or sensory innervation to the bladder and bowel.

Where is lumbar intervertebral disc herniation most common?

Between L_4 and L_5 or between L_5 and S_1 (Figure 6.5).

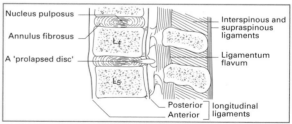

FIGURE 6.5 – Intervertebral disk herniation.

What happens to the turgor strength of the nucleus pulposus as people age?

Dehydration and degeneration cause this structure to lose its large water content (decreasing turgor) and facilitates herniation.

What is the most frequent direction of nucleus pulposus herniation?

Posterolateral (primarily due to a hyperflexion injury).

Does typical herniation of the nucleus pulposus directly compress the spinal cord?

No. The cauda equina is posterior to the intervertebral (IV) discs at the most common levels of disc herniation. The neurologic symptoms are a result of spinal nerve impingement.

Which IV disc is responsible for compression of the L₅ spinal nerve when it herniates?

The IV disc between L_4 and L_5.

If a radiograph shows the forward slippage of one vertebral body over the vertebral body directly below it, what is the most likely diagnosis?

Spondylolisthesis (Figure 6.6).

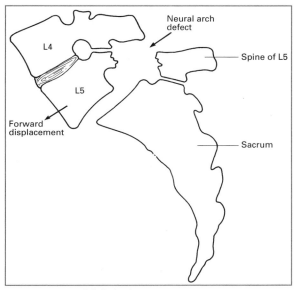

FIGURE 6.6 – Spondylolisthesis.

What is spondylolysis?

A fracture and separation of the pars inter-articularis of the vertebral arch. Spondylolysis can eventually lead to spondylolisthesis.

 Memory Aid: Spondylo**lysis** versus spondylolisthesis: **lysis** refers to the fracture.

What is the classic radiographic finding in spondylolysis?

A collar around the neck of the Scotty dog.

What is the most common reason for performing a lumbar puncture?

Altered mental status for quick and safe evaluation of meningitis and subarachnoid hemorrhages.

What is the typical vertebral level and bony landmark used in performing lumbar punctures in adults?

Between L_4 and L_5, at the level of the iliac crests. In adults, the spinal cord ends at L_1 or L_2, and thus, a lumbar puncture may be performed at the L_3–L_4 interspace as well.

List the layers that are pierced when accessing the cerebrospinal fluid (in the subarachnoid space).

Skin and superficial fascia, supraspinous ligament, interspinous ligament, ligamentum flavum, dura mater, subdural space, arachnoid, and subarachnoid space (Figure 6.7).

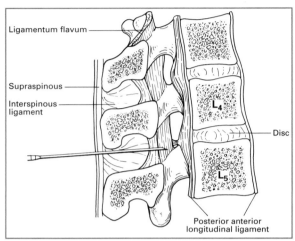

FIGURE 6.7 – Lumbar puncture.

OSTEOPATHIC PRINCIPLES

What are the three planes of motion for the lumbar spine?

1. Flexion and extension in the sagittal plane.
2. Sidebending (lateral flexion) in the coronal plane.
3. Rotation in the transverse (horizontal) plane.

What is the primary motion exhibited by lumbar spine?

Flexion and extension. Then, lateral flexion > rotation.

What types of somatic dysfunction can be found in the lumbar spine?

Lumbar somatic dysfunctions may be group curves (type I somatic dysfunction) or single somatic dysfunction (type II somatic dysfunction). In the lumbar spine, group curves are more common.

(See Chapter 4: Thoracic for type I & II somatic dysfunction.)

What are two major causes of lumbar group curves?

Thoracic spine scoliosis and sacral base unleveling.

What is the Ferguson's (lumbosacral) angle?

The angle of inclination, above the horizontal plane, of the sacral base (where L_5 meets S_1) (Figure 6.8).

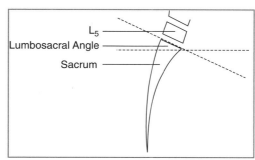

FIGURE 6.8 – Lumbosacral angle.

What organs/regions do the following pre-ganglionic sympathetic nerves innervate?

T10–L2	**Prostate and prostatic urethra (in males).** **Uterus and cervix (in females).**
T11–L2	**Lower extremity.**
T12–L1	**Lower ureter.**
T12–L2	**Hindgut (up to the pectinate line), bladder.**
L1–L2	**Distal $\frac{1}{3}$ of transverse colon, descending colon, sigmoid colon, and rectum.**

DIAGNOSIS

What primary observations should be made when examining the lumbar spine?

1. Erythema (blanching)
2. Skin temperature
3. Skin texture
4. Skin moisture or dryness
5. Muscle spasm
6. Scars
7. Lordosis (increased/decreased)
8. Lateral curves

How is dynamic motion testing for the lumbar spine performed?

With examiner's thumbs on the transverse processes of the lumbar vertebra, the standing patient is asked to bend forward and then backward to test flexion and extension, respectively. The patient can then be asked to twist to both sides above the waist to check rotation and bend side-to-side to assess lateral flexion.

Remember: Somatic dysfunctions are named for their freedoms, i.e., the direction in which greater motion is palpated.

How is static testing of the lumbar spine performed?

Patient is seated or prone. Examiner places thumbs over transverse processes of vertebra being diagnosed. By rolling thumbs to superior edge of transverse processes and applying pressure, flexion can be assessed. Similarly, by rolling thumbs to inferior edge of transverse processes, extension is assessed. The vertebra can then be translated to both sides to assess sidebending. Translation to one side tests sidebending to the contralateral side (e.g., left translation is coupled with right sidebending). Rotation can be assessed by applying pressure anteriorly on one transverse process and then the opposite one.

SPECIAL TESTS

What is the Thomas' test?

See Chapter 10: Lower Extremity—Special Tests.

The Thomas' test is for the iliopsoas m. How does this muscle affect the lumbar spine?

A flexion contracture of the iliopsoas m. (positive Thomas' test result) can increase the lordosis of the lumbar spine because the psoas m. attachments span across the lumbar spine. This makes the lumbar spine more vulnerable to low back pain, degenerative joint disease, disc herniation, spondylolisthesis, spondylolysis, etc.

TREATMENT

What are the direct effects of treatment of lumbar spine somatic dysfunctions?

↑ back range of motion, normalize sympathetic outflow, ↓ muscle spasms, ↓ fascial strains, ↓ ligamentous tension, change center of gravity location, improved diaphragm function, and improved hip motion.

What are specific contraindications to high velocity low amplitude (HVLA) of the lumbar vertebra?

Aside from the contraindications mentioned in Chapter 1, those specific to the lumbar vertebrae when using HVLA include abdominal aortic aneurysm, abdominal cavity wound/trauma, vertebral fracture, spondylolysis, spondylolisthesis, and herniated disc (relative).

What are the general rules for counterstrain (CS) treatments of the lumbar spine?

Anterior CS tenderpoints require flexion and posterior tenderpoints require extension (Figure 6.9).

Remember: Lower Pole L_5 is an exception to this rule.

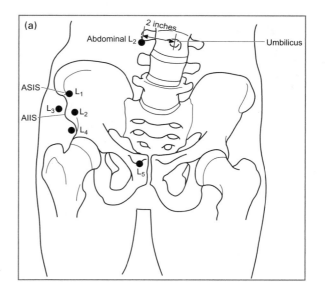

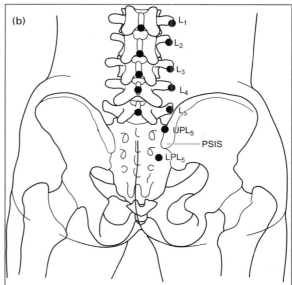

FIGURE 6.9 – A: Anterior lumbar tenderpoints. B: Posterior lumbar tenderpoints. UPL$_5$ – Upper Pole L$_5$; LPL$_5$ – Lower Pole L$_5$.

How is the tenderpoint of lower pole L$_5$ treated with counterstrain?

Patient is prone and ipsilateral leg is dropped off the side of table. The hip and knee are flexed and then used to induce internal rotation and adduction at the hip.

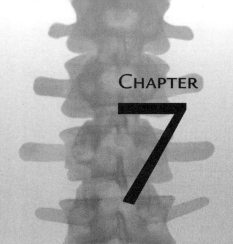

CHAPTER 7 INNOMINATES

GROSS ANATOMY OVERVIEW

What forms the pelvic girdle?	The pelvic girdle is formed by the pubic bones meeting anteriorly and the sacrum joining the innominates posteriorly.
Where do all the bones of each innominate converge?	In the acetabulum.

Identify the bony landmarks on the innominates (Figure 7.1):

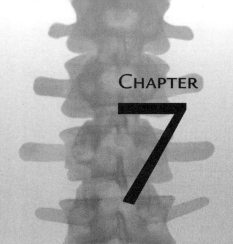

1. Posterior superior iliac spine (PSIS)
2. Posterior inferior iliac spine
3. Greater sciatic notch
4. Ischial spine
5. Lesser sciatic notch
6. Obturator foramen
7. Ischial tuberosity
8. Iliac crest
9. Anterior superior iliac spine (ASIS)
10. Anterior inferior iliac spine
11. Acetabulum
12. Superior pubic ramus
13. Pubic tubercle
14. Inferior pubic ramus.

FIGURE 7.1 – Innominate osteology.

Describe the iliac crest.	The thick superior rim of the ilium.
Where is the ASIS?	The most anterior projection of the iliac crest.
Where is the PSIS?	The most posterior projection of the iliac crest.
What is the large infero-posterior protuberance of the ischium?	Ischial tuberosity (it's the bony part you sit on).
Name the foramen in either innominate enclosed by the ischium and pubis.	Obturator foramen.

Define the pelvic inlet.

It is the spatial plane passing through the superior margin of the pubic symphysis and the sacral promontory (Figure 7.2).

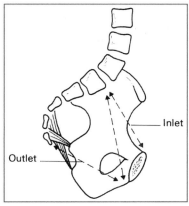

FIGURE 7.2 – Pelvic inlet and outlet.

Define the pelvic outlet.

It is the spatial plane passing through the inferior margin of the pubic symphysis and the tip of the coccyx (see Figure 7.2).

Where is the greater pelvis?

The pelvic region above the pelvic inlet (A.K.A. false pelvis or pelvis major).

Where is the lesser pelvis?

The pelvic region between the pelvic inlet and outlet (A.K.A. true pelvis or pelvis minor).

List all the ligaments connecting the vertebral column with the ilium.

1. Iliolumbar ligaments
2. Posterior sacroiliac ligaments
3. Anterior sacroiliac ligaments.

What are the names of the ligaments between the ischium and the sacrum?

1. Sacrospinous ligament
2. Sacrotuberous ligament.

What foramen does the sacrospinous ligaments create?

The greater sciatic foramen (Figure 7.3).

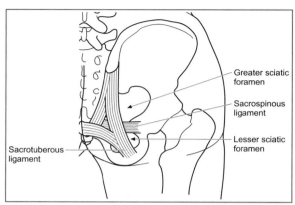

FIGURE 7.3 – Sciatic foramina.

What are the boundaries of the lesser sciatic foramen?

1. Sacrospinous ligament
2. Sacrotuberous ligament
3. Ischium.

What muscles make up the pelvic diaphragm?

1. Puborectalis mm. (antero-medial levator ani m.)
2. Pubococcygeus mm. (levator ani group)
3. Iliococcygeus mm. (postero-lateral levator ani m.)
4. Ischiococcygeus mm. (A.K.A. coccygeus mm.) (Figure 7.4).

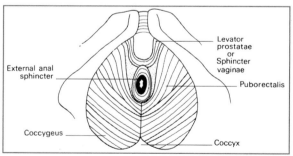

FIGURE 7.4 – Pelvic diaphragm.

What are the attachments of the levator ani mm.?

1. Body of pubis
2. Tendinous arch of obturator fascia
3. Ischial spine
4. Perineal body
5. Coccyx
6. Anococcygeal ligament
7. Walls of prostate, vagina, rectum, and anal canal.

What is the innervation of the levator ani mm.?	Nerve to levator ani (branch of S<u>4</u> nerve ventral ramus), inferior rectal n., and coccygeal plexus. **Memory Aid:** S<u>4</u> for all <u>4</u> levator ani mm.
What is the "central tendon" of the pelvic diaphragm?	Perineal body.
Name the structures that traverse the pelvic diaphragm.	Vagina, prostate, urethra, anal canal, neurovascular bundles, and lymphatics.

CLINICAL ANATOMY

During pregnancy, what anatomic changes will help to increase the transverse diameter of the pelvis and facilitate passage of the fetus?	Hormonal relaxation (relaxin) of the sacroiliac joints and nutation/counternutation of the sacrum.
List the four types of pelvic shapes.	1. Gynecoid 2. Android 3. Anthropoid 4. Platypelloid (Figure 7.5).

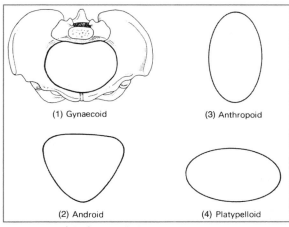

(1) Gynaecoid (3) Anthropoid

(2) Android (4) Platypelloid

FIGURE 7.5 – Pelvic shape variations.

List the functions of the pelvic diaphragm.	1. Support pelvic viscera 2. Allows and compensates for changes in intra-abdominal pressure (for respiration and blood and lymphatic flow) 3. Pulls coccyx anteriorly (sacrococcygeal mobility) 4. Weight-bearing 5. Anal continence (via puborectal sling).

List the four weak areas of the pelvis where fractures are most likely to occur.	1. Pubic rami 2. Acetabula 3. Sacroiliac joint 4. Alae of the ilium.
What is a tri-radiate cartilage fracture?	A fracture through the ossifying acetabular cartilage in persons younger than 17 years old, dividing the acetabulum into ilial, ischial, and pubic fragments.

OSTEOPATHIC PRINCIPLES

What is the function of the pelvic girdle?	• Resists stress • Transmits load between the vertebral column and lower limb.
What major landmarks are used to ascertain motion of the innominates?	Three: 1. ASIS 2. PSIS 3. Pubic tubercles. *Remember: You can use hand models corresponding to these three landmarks to figure out innominate somatic dysfunctions (Figure 7.6).*

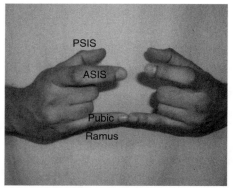

FIGURE 7.6 – Hand model of innominates.

List the motions of the ilia on the sacrum.	1. Anterior/posterior rotation 2. Inflare and outflare 3. Superior/inferior translation 4. Anterior/posterior translation.

Where is the axis for anterior/posterior rotation of the ilia?

Inferior transverse axis of sacrum; passes horizontally through the inferior pole of the sacro-iliac articulation (level through S_3 or S_4) (Figure 7.7).

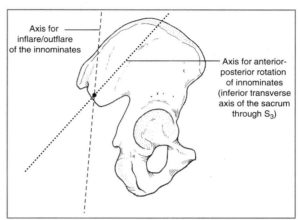

FIGURE 7.7 – Axes of innominate motion.

What is the axis for inflare/outflare motion of ilia?

Imaginary longitudinal line that passes through the sacro-iliac joint (see Figure 7.7).

List the pubic motions at their symphysis.

Three (Figure 7.8):

1. Caliper
2. Torsion (horizontal axis through the pubic bones)
3. Translation (superior/inferior/anterior/posterior).

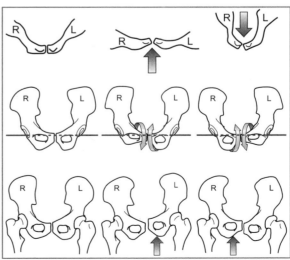

FIGURE 7.8 – Pubic motions.

Describe the motion of the innominate during stance phase of normal gait.	Starting with heel-strike, the ipsilateral innominate shifts superiorly and rotates anteriorly until toe-off.
What motion of the innominate is associated with the swing phase leg of normal gait?	Starting with toe-off, the ipsilateral innominate shifts inferiorly and rotates posteriorly on the side of the swing leg. (These motions compliment the motions coupled with the stance leg.)

DIAGNOSIS

What are signs and symptoms associated with innominate dysfunction?	Back, hip, groin, and knee pain; pain radiating to lower extremity (LE); difficulty walking/limping; and local tenderness, edema, and erythema.
What is the purpose of the standing flexion test?	**To assess iliosacral function, a positive test result is seen with innominate dysfunction. This test helps the examiner determine which side is dysfunctional (innominate findings should be recorded on this side).**
How is the standing flexion test performed?	Patient stands erect with feet shoulder width apart. Examiner monitors PSIS bilaterally with thumbs, allowing fingers to rest on the iliac crests. Patient is instructed to bend forward (flex) slowly reaching for their toes while keeping the legs straight.
What is a positive standing flexion test result?	The side with greater superior displacement of the PSIS (monitored by examiner's thumb).
What does a positive standing flexion test result indicate?	It indicates innominate dysfunction. When the patient bends forward, the sacrum flexes. In the presence of innominate dysfunction, the ipsilateral iliosacral joint locks prematurely and causes the PSIS to follow the sacrum superiorly.
What is a false-negative standing flexion test result?	**When there is a bilateral innominate dysfunction, both PSIS move superiorly along with the sacrum, making it difficult to distinguish just one side as dysfunctional.**
How can tight hamstring mm. affect the results of a standing flexion test?	**Tight hamstrings may not allow for free anterior rotation of the innominates as the patient bends forward during the standing flexion test, resulting in false results.**
What is another method to assess iliosacral motion?	The ASIS compression test: by compressing the ASIS medially, one can assess motion at the iliosacral joint. A restriction to ASIS compression would indicate ipsilateral innominate dysfunction.

Describe the following innominate dysfunctions:	*Note: An innominate rotation, an innominate shear, an innominate flare, and pubic shear may occur concomitantly. (See Figure 7.6 on hand models and dysfunctions.)*
Anterior innominate/ilial rotation	The ASIS is inferior and the PSIS is superior on the side of the positive standing flexion test.
Posterior innominate/ilial rotation	Ipsilateral findings: • Positive standing flexion test result • ASIS is superior • PSIS is inferior.
Superior innominate/ilial shear	Ipsilateral findings: • Positive standing flexion test result • ASIS is superior • PSIS is superior • Pubic tubercle is superior.
Inferior innominate/ilial shear	Ipsilateral findings: • Positive standing flexion test result • ASIS is inferior • PSIS is inferior • Pubic tubercle is inferior.
Ilial inflare	On the side of the positive standing flexion test result, the ipsilateral ASIS is closer to the umbilicus than the contralateral ASIS.
Ilial outflare	On the side of the positive standing flexion test result, the ipsilateral ASIS is further from the umbilicus than the contralateral ASIS.
Superior pubic shear	The pubic tubercle is superior on the same side as the positive standing flexion test result.
Inferior pubic shear	The pubic tubercle is inferior on the same side as the positive standing flexion test result.
How do innominate dysfunctions affect leg length?	**Function/dysfunction of the innominates can affect the location of the acetabulum, in turn affecting the distal LE.**
Which innominate somatic dysfunction may present as a short leg? How?	Innominate somatic dysfunctions that cause the acetabulum to displace superiorly. These include: 1. Posterior innominate/ilial rotation 2. Superior innominate/ilial shear
Which innominate somatic dysfunction may present as a long leg? How?	Innominate somatic dysfunctions that cause the acetabulum to displace inferiorly. These include: 1. Anterior innominate/ilial rotation 2. Inferior innominate/ilial shear

SPECIAL TESTS

What is the standing flexion test?	See previous section.
What is the ASIS compression test?	See previous section.
How does one perform the stork test?	Patient is standing in front of examiner. Examiner places thumbs over patient's PSIS bilaterally. Patient is asked to flex the hip and knee to 90 degrees each one leg at a time with the other leg straight. Note motion of the PSIS.
Describe a positive stork test result.	The side with lesser posterior/inferior motion of the PSIS is the side of iliosacral locking and thus, the side of the somatic dysfunction.
What does a positive Erichsen's test result indicate?	Sacroiliac disease, generally involving a form of degenerative joint disease in this area, especially early spondylitic arthritis.
How does one perform an Erichsen's test?	Patient is supine, examiner's hands over lateral aspect of ilial alae bilaterally. Examiner compresses medially. Positive test is indicated by pain (Figure 7.9).

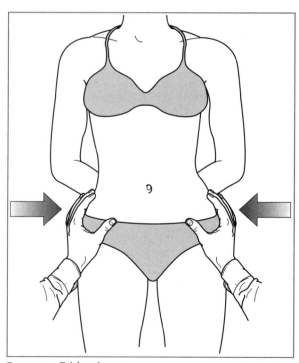

FIGURE 7.9 – Erichsen's test.

How does the FAbERE (Patrick's) test screen sacroiliac joint pathology?	To learn how to perform the FAbERE test, *see Chapter 10: Lower Extremity—Special Tests*. The motion of this test compresses the sacroiliac joint and can thus screen sacroiliac disease.

TREATMENT

What can treatment of the innominates affect?	Gait, back pain, hip pain, knee pain, spasms of muscles attached to innominates, leg length, hip/sacroiliac (SI) range of motion.
Which treatment modalities can be used in innominate treatment?	Facilitated positional release, muscle energy, high velocity low amplitude, balanced ligamentous tension, ligamentous articular strain, and myofascial are commonly used techniques when treating the innominates.
Treatment of what joint improves innominate somatic dysfunction?	SI joint
How can the SI joint be treated?	SI joint release: Examiner places fingers along the SI joint and distracts the innominates laterally away from the sacrum. By distracting the ischial tuberosity simultaneously, one can also perform a pelvic hemi-diaphragm release.
What are the direct effects of treatment of the pelvic diaphragm?	↑ Lymphatic and vascular flow from lower extremities/pelvis, ↑ abdominal/pelvic compensation for respiration, improve urethral position/function, improve fecal continence, improve vaginal function, ↓ vaginal discomfort.
How is the pelvic diaphragm treated?	Patient may be supine with hip and knees flexed or prone. Examiner will push superiorly on the pelvic diaphragm just medial to the ischial tuberosities bilaterally. Treatment may be improved with lateral traction of the ischial tuberosities.
How can respiratory assist be used in pelvic diaphragm release?	Perform the pelvic diaphragm release as above; however, when the patient inhales, resist inferior motion of pelvic diaphragm. When the patient exhales, exaggerate the superior motion of the pelvic diaphragm.

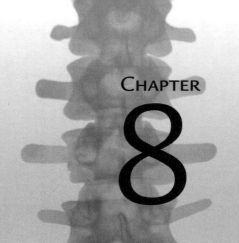

GROSS ANATOMY OVERVIEW

Dermatomes from the Sacral Spine (Figure 8.1)

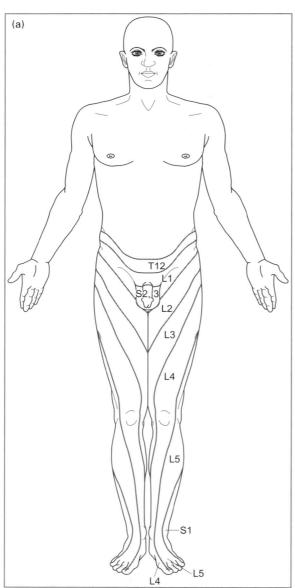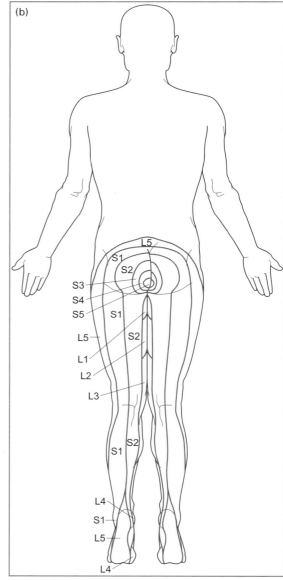

FIGURE 8.1 – Dermatomes from the sacral spine.

Sacral Osteology (Figure 8.2)

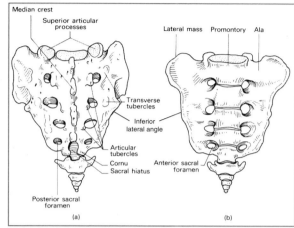

FIGURE 8.2 – Sacral osteology.

Surface Anatomy of the Sacrum (Figure 8.3)

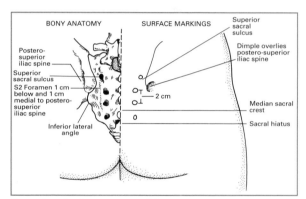

FIGURE 8.3 – Surface anatomy of the sacrum.

How many vertebrae fuse to create the sacrum? The coccyx?	Five vertebrae fuse to form the sacrum. Four rudimentary vertebrae fuse to form the coccyx.
When does fusion of the sacral vertebrae begin?	After the 20th year of life.
What part of the central nervous system can be found in the sacral canal?	Cauda equina (nerve roots within the meninges) and filum terminale (pia mater extension from the conus medullaris).
What is the anterior projection of the S_1 vertebra called?	Sacral promontory (used to make measurements of the pelvic inlet).
What major hip muscle originates from the sacrum?	Piriformis m.

CLINICAL ANATOMY

What are the bony landmarks for performing caudal epidural anesthesia?

Sacral hiatus between the sacral cornua (inferior to the 4th sacral spinous process) (Figure 8.4).

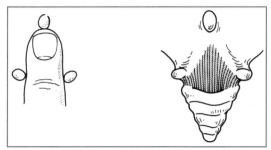

FIGURE 8.4 – Sacral hiatus.

What spinal nerves are affected by caudal anesthesia?

Local anesthetic acts on S2 through coccygeal spinal nerves and sensation is lost inferior to this epidural block (Figure 8.5).

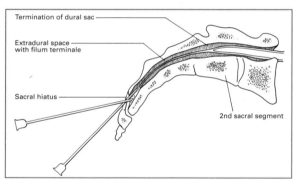

FIGURE 8.5 – Caudal anesthesia.

What is the term for an L_5 vertebra partially or completely fused with the sacrum?

Sacralization.

What is lumbarization?

S_1 vertebra separated from sacrum and partially or completely fused with L_5.

OSTEOPATHIC PRINCIPLES

What is the sacroiliac (SI) joint?

The joint where the sacrum moves relative to the ilium. When observing motion of the ilium relative to the sacrum, the same articulation between the sacrum and ilium is referred to as the iliosacral joint.

How many axes guide sacral motion?

Seven (Figure 8.6).

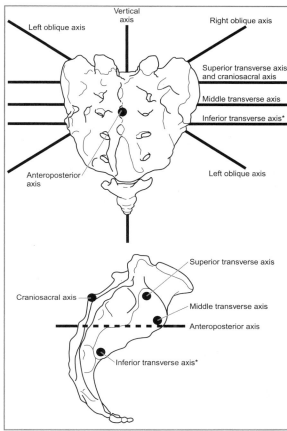

FIGURE 8.6 – Axes of sacral motion.

* The inferior transverse axis, though it passes through the sacrum, defines anterior and posterior rotational motion of the innominates. (See Chapter 7: Innominates—Osteopathic Principles for more information.)

What are the different types of motion exhibited by the sacrum?

1. Craniosacral motion (flexion/extension)— Craniosacral axis of sacrum

2. Respiratory motion and cranial motion— Superior transverse axis

3. Postural/structural motion (flexion/extension) —Middle transverse axis

4. Torsion (dynamic) motion—Left oblique axis and/or right oblique axis

5. Rotation (left/right)—Vertical axis

6. Lateral flexion (left/right)—Anteroposterior axis.

How many transverse axes pass through S_2? Name them.	Two transverse axes pass through S_2: 1. Superior transverse axis (anterior to spinal canal) 2. Craniosacral axis (posterior to spinal canal) *Note: For purposes of the boards, it is important to know the superior transverse axis and craniosacral axis, both, pass through S_2. Many sources consider them to be one axis allowing both respiratory and craniosacral flexion/extension.*
Describe postural (structural) flexion and extension of the sacrum.	Postural flexion and extension of the sacrum occurs around the middle transverse axis of the sacrum. During sacral postural flexion, the base of the sacrum moves anterior. During sacral postural extension, the base of the sacrum moves posterior. *Remember: Postural flexion/extension of the sacrum is similar to vertebral flexion/extension. Think of the sacrum as one giant vertebra → during flexion the superior aspect moves anterior and during extension, the superior portion moves posterior.*
How is cranial motion of the sacrum different from postural motion?	1. **Separate axes of motion: The axis for cranial motion is posterior to the spinal canal through the superior articular pillars of S_2, whereas, the axis for postural motion is through S_3 (middle transverse axis).** 2. **Cranial motion of the sacrum is opposite to structural motion, i.e., cranial flexion involves posterior motion of the sacral base and cranial extension is anterior motion of the sacral base.** *Note: When the type (postural or cranial) of flexion/ extension is not specified, the motion described is assumed to be postural.*
Describe the motion of the sacrum with respiration.	**Respiration engages motion at the superior transverse axis of the sacrum. With inspiration (as the respiratory diaphragm lowers and the abdominal pressure increases), the base of the sacrum moves posterior. During exhalation (respiratory diaphragm rises and abdominal pressure decreases), the sacral base moves anterior.**
When are the oblique axes engaged during physiologic motion of the sacrum?	During gait, the oblique axis on the side of the stance leg is engaged. For example, during normal gait, when the left leg is the stance leg, the left oblique axis is engaged.
Is an anterior sacral sulcus considered deep or shallow upon palpation?	Deep.

*What is the difference between an **inferior** and **posterior** inferior lateral angle (ILA)?*

Motion of the ILA is coupled—when the ILA moves posteriorly, it also moves inferiorly. Thus, when an ILA is noted to be inferior, it can be assumed that it is posterior as well.

What organs/regions do the pre-ganglionic parasympathetic nerves from the sacrum innervate?

Gastrointestinal tract distal to ⅔ transverse colon, distal ureters, urinary bladder, prostate/uterus, and genitalia.

DIAGNOSIS

What primary observations should be made when examining the sacrum?

1. Erythema (blanching)
2. Skin temperature
3. Skin texture/hair over sacrum
4. Skin moisture or dryness
5. Scars
6. Lumbar lordosis (increased/decreased).

What is a best screening test for sacral somatic dysfunction?

The seated flexion test. See special tests below to learn how to perform the seated flexion test.

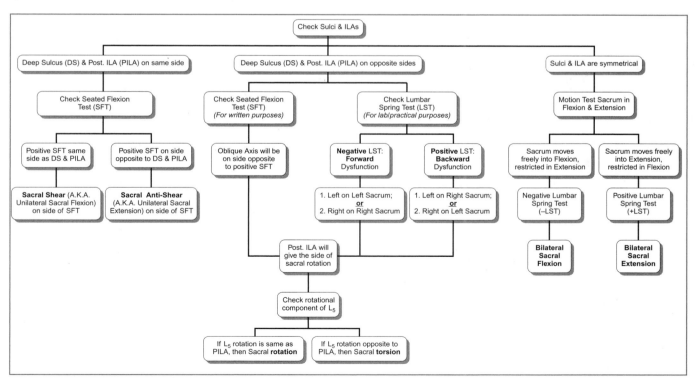

FIGURE 8.7 – Sacrum diagnosis algorithm.

What is the first step when diagnosing somatic dysfunction of the sacrum?

Always check the sacral sulci (which one is deeper and/or anterior) and ILAs (which one is more posterior or inferior).

If the deep (anterior) sulcus and the posterior (or inferior) ILA are both on the same side, what type of sacral somatic dysfunction may be present?

Unilateral sacral flexion (A.K.A. sacral shear) or unilateral sacral extension (A.K.A. sacral anti-shear)

*What is a **unilateral sacral flexion** (A.K.A. sacral shear)?*

One side of the **sacrum** (**unilaterally** on the side of the positive seated flexion test) is free to move into **flexion** however restricted in extension. The opposite side is free to move in both flexion and extension (Figure 8.8A).

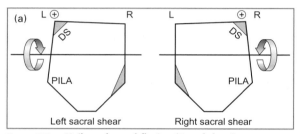

FIGURE 8.8A – Unilateral sacral flexion (Sacral shear).
⊕: Positive seated flexion test; DS: Deep (anterior) sulcus; PILA: Posterior (inferior) I.L.A.

*What is a **unilateral sacral extension** (A.K.A. sacral anti-shear)?*

One side of the **sacrum** (**unilaterally** on the side of the positive seated flexion test) is free to move into **extension** however restricted in flexion. The opposite side is free to move in both flexion and extension (Figure 8.8B).

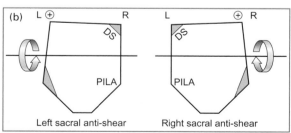

FIGURE 8.8B – Unilateral sacral extension (sacral anti-shear).
⊕: Positive seated flexion test; DS: Deep (anterior) sulcus; PILA: Posterior (inferior) I.L.A.

What are the two possible forward sacral dysfunctions?

1. Right rotation on right oblique axis forward sacral dysfunction (R on R sacral dysfxn)

2. Left rotation on left oblique axis forward sacral dysfunction (L on L sacral dysfxn) (Figure 8.8C).

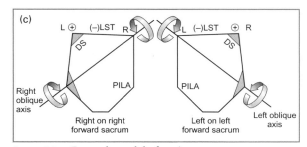

FIGURE 8.8c – Forward sacral dysfunctions.
⊕: Positive seated flexion test; DS: Deep (anterior) sulcus; PILA: Posterior (inferior) I.L.A.; (–)LST: Negative lumbar spring test; (+)LST: Positive lumbar spring test.

What are the two possible backward sacral dysfunctions?

1. Right rotation on left oblique axis forward sacral dysfunction (R on L sacral dysfxn)

2. Left rotation on right oblique axis forward sacral dysfunction (L on R sacral dysfxn) (Figure 8.8D).

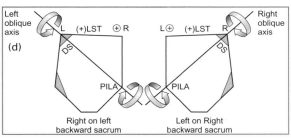

FIGURE 8.8D – Backward sacral dysfunctions.
⊕: Positive seated flexion test; DS: Deep (anterior) sulcus; PILA: Posterior (inferior) I.L.A.; (–)LST: Negative lumbar spring test; (+)LST: Positive lumbar spring test.

What is the difference between a forward sacral dysfunction and a backward sacral dysfunction?

In a forward sacral dysfunction, the base of the sacrum is free to move anterior (into sacral flexion) and the rotation and oblique axis of the sacrum are on the same side.

In a backward sacral dysfunction, the base of the sacrum is free to move posterior (into sacral extension) and the rotation and oblique axis of the sacrum are on opposite sides.

What is the difference between a sacral rotation and a sacral torsion?

In a sacral **rotation**, the sacrum and L_5 are **both rotated** to the **same side**.

In a sacral **torsion**, the sacrum and L_5 are rotated to **opposite sides**, creating a **twist** at the lumbosacral junction.

What is a **bilateral sacral flexion**?

Both sides of the sacrum (**bilaterally**) are capable of moving into **flexion** (remember dysfunctions are named for their freedoms) but restricted in extension (Figure 8.8E).

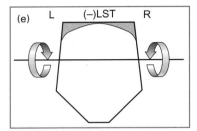

FIGURE 8.8E – Bilateral sacral flexion.
(−)LST: Negative lumbar spring test; (+)LST: Positive lumbar spring test.

What is a **bilateral sacral extension**?

Both sides of the sacrum (**bilaterally**) are capable of moving into **extension** but restricted in flexion (Figure 8.8F).

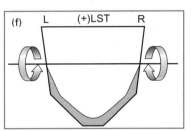

FIGURE 8.8F – Bilateral sacral extension.
(−)LST: Negative lumbar spring test; (+)LST: Positive lumbar spring test.

SPECIAL TESTS

How is the seated flexion (forward-bending) test performed?

The patient is seated with hips and knees flexed 90 degrees and both feet flat on the floor. The examiner places his thumbs over the patient's posterior superior iliac spine (PSIS) bilaterally and asks the patient to touch the floor with his hands. Care must be taken that the patient is not resting his arms on his thighs during the test.

What is a positive seated flexion test result?

The side on which the PSIS (monitored by examiner's thumb) displaces further superiorly.

What does a positive seated flexion test result indicate?	When the patient bends forward, the sacrum flexes forward relative to the innominate, which is stabilized by the ischial tuberosity (because the patient is sitting). In the presence of innominate dysfunction, the SI joint locks prematurely and causes the PSIS to follow the sacrum superiorly. Any such SI locking is indicative of sacral dysfunction. Thus the seated flexion can serve as an excellent general screening test for sacral dysfunction.
Can more specific information be derived from the seated flexion test?	Yes, depending on the findings at the sacral sulci and ILAs, the seated flexion test can provide more specific information:

1. Seated flexion test, deep (anterior) sulcus and posterior (inferior) ILA are all on the same side—A unilateral sacral flexion exists on the same side as the seated flexion test.
2. Seated flexion test is on opposite side of the deep sulcus and posterior ILA—A unilateral sacral extension exists on the same side as the seated flexion test.
3. Deep sulcus and posterior ILA are on opposite sides of each other—The oblique axis of rotation will be on the side opposite to the positive seated flexion test (see Figure 8.7).

*What is a **false**-negative seated flexion test result?*	When there is a bilateral sacral dysfunction, **both PSIS move superiorly** along with the sacrum, making it difficult to distinguish just any one side as dysfunctional.
*What is a **false**-positive seated flexion test result?*	Spasm of muscles such as the quadratus lumborum, latissimus dorsi, and psoas that attach to the upper torso and innominates/hip can cause the innominates to rotate anteriorly as the patient bends forward and give the appearance of a positive seated flexion test result.
How is the lumbar spring test performed?	The patient is asked to lay prone. The examiner places hand midline over L_4 to S_1. Pressure is applied straight down toward the table to check whether the lumbosacral junction springs forward or resists anterior motion.

*What is a **positive** lumbar spring test result?*	When **no** anterior motion can be produced at the lumbosacral junction. Thus, there is no springing possible in a positive lumbar spring test result. Patients with a flattened or kyphotic lumbar spine are likely to have a positive lumbar spring test.
What can be concluded from a negative lumbar spring test result?	1. **Lumbar lordosis is normal or increased. (This also implies the lumbar spine is free to move in extension. However, this does not mean there is a restriction in flexion!)** 2. **Sacral base prefers Forward (anterior) motion such as in sacral Flexion.**
What conclusions can be drawn from a positive lumbar spring test?	1. **Lumbar spine is flattened or kyphotic. (This implies the lumbar spine is restricted in extension.)** 2. **Sacral base prefers backward (posterior) motion such as in sacral extension.**
How is the sphinx (A.K.A. backward-bending) test performed?	Patient is prone or standing. Examiner places thumbs over the sacral sulci and makes note of their depth. Patient is asked to extend the lumbar spine by lifting upper torso off table using elbows (sphinx or TV position) or by bending/leaning backward at the waist.
What is a positive sphinx test result?	Lack of anterior motion (deepening) of either sacral sulcus.
What does a positive sphinx test result signify?	Extension of the lumbar spine causes the base of sacrum to move anterior (flexion). A positive sphinx test result indicates there is an SI motion (flexion) restriction on the side of the positive test result.

TREATMENT

What are the direct effects of treatment of sacral somatic dysfunctions?	↑ back and hip range of motion, normalize parasympathetic outflow, ↓ fascial strains, ↓ ligamentous tension, improved pelvic diaphragm function, and improved hip motion.
What is the role of L_5 in sacral somatic dysfunction?	**Motion of the sacrum can be related to L_5. Therefore, when somatic dysfunction is found at L_5, sacral dysfunction will be present. Also, to complete treatment of the sacrum, L_5 must be treated.**

Anterior and Posterior Sacral Tenderpoints
(Figure 8.9)

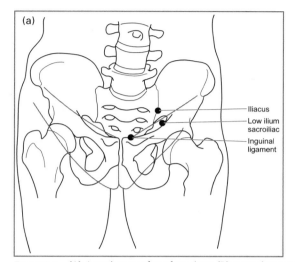
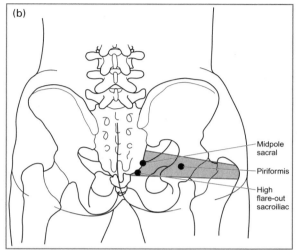

FIGURE 8.9 – (A) Anterior sacral tenderpoints; (B) posterior sacral tenderpoints.
     *The posterior sacral tenderpoints overlie the piriformis m., shown as the shaded area in figure 8.9 (B).

SECTION III

Extremities

GROSS ANATOMY OVERVIEW

Dermatomes of the Upper Extremity (Figure 9.1)

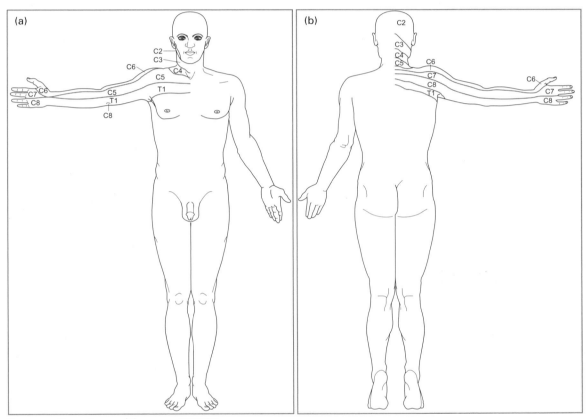

FIGURE 9.1 – Dermatomes of the upper extremity.

TABLE 9.1 – **Range of Motion of Upper Extremity Joints**

Joint	Motion	Range (in degrees)
Shoulder	Flexion	0–180
	Extension	0–60
	Abduction	0–180
	Adduction	0–70
	External rotation	0–70
	Internal rotation	0–90
Elbow	Flexion	0–150
	Extension	0°
	Supination (of forearm)	0–90
	Pronation (of forearm)	0–90
Wrist	Flexion	0–80
	Extension	0–70
	Ulnar (medial) deviation	0–30
	Radial (lateral) deviation	0–20

Identify the nerves exitting the brachial plexus in Figure 9.2.
Answers are in Table 9.2.

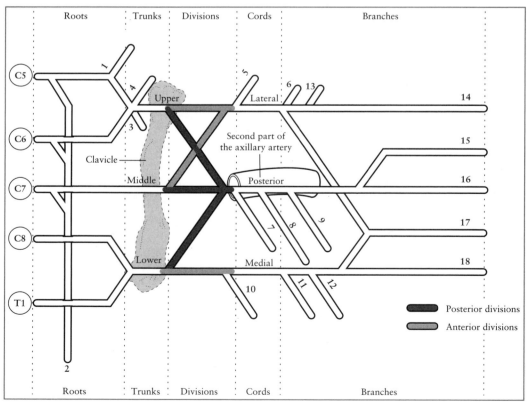

FIGURE 9.2 – Brachial plexus.

TABLE 9.2 – **Brachial Plexus**

No.	Nerve	Innervation
1	Dorsal scapular n. (C5)	Rhomboids (major and minor) mm., Levator scapulae m.
2	Long thoracic n. (C5, C6, C7)	Serratus anterior m.
3	N. to subclavius (C5, C6)	Subclavius m.
4	Suprascapular n. (C5, C6)	Supraspinatus m., Infraspinatus m.
5	Lateral pectoral n. (C5, C6, C7)	Pectoralis major m.
6	Lateral brachial cutaneous nn. (C5, C6, C7)	Sensory innervation of the lateral aspect of arm. Upper lateral brachial cutaneous n. is a branch of the axillary n. Lower lateral brachial cutaneous n. is a branch of the radial n.
7	Upper subscapular n. (C5, C6)	Superior portion of subscapularis m.
8	Thoracodorsal (middle subscapular) n. (C6, C7, C8)	Latissimus dorsi m.
9	Lower subscapular n. (C5, C6)	Inferior portion of subscapularis m. and teres major m.
10	Medial pectoral n. (C8, T1)	Pectoralis major and minor mm.
11	Medial brachial cutaneous n. (C8, T1)	Sensory innervation of the medial aspect of arm
12	Medial antebrachial cutaneous n. (C8, T1)	Sensory innervation of the medial aspect of forearm
13	Lateral antebrachial cutaneous n. (C5, C6, C7)	Sensory innervation of the lateral aspect of forearm
14	Musculocutaneous n. (C5, C6, C7)	Coracobrachialis m., Biceps brachii m., Brachialis m.
15	Axillary n. (C5, C6)	Deltoid m., Teres minor m.
16	Radial n. (C5, C6, C7, C8, T1)	Triceps brachii m., anconeus m., brachioradialis m., all extensor mm. of elbow and forearm, abductor pollicis longus m.
17	Median n. (C6, C7, C8, T1)	Pronator teres m., palmaris longus m., flexor carpi radialis m., flexor digitorum superficialis m., flexor digitorum profundus m. (radial half), flexor pollicis longus m., first and second lumbrical mm., opponens pollicis m., abductor pollicis brevis m., flexor pollicis brevis m.
18	Ulnar n. (C8, T1)	Flexor carpi ulnaris m., flexor digitorum profundus m. (ulnar half), adductor pollicis m., third and fourth lumbrical mm., palmar and dorsal interossei mm., opponens digiti minimi m., flexor digiti minimi m., abductor digiti minimi m., adductor digiti minimi m.

Memory Aid: Median n.

Forearm—All flexors of the **forearm** except flexor carpi ulnaris m. and ulnar half of flexor digitorum profundus m. are innervated by the median n.

Hand—First and second (**two**) **L**umbrical mm., **O**pponens pollicis m., **A**bductor pollicis brevis m., **F**lexor pollicis brevis m.—**2 LOAF**.

TABLE 9.3 – **Upper Extremity Muscles**

Name of Muscle	Origin	Insertion	Action
Trapezius m.	Superior nuchal line, ligamentum nuchae and spinous process (SP) of C_1 to T_{12}.	Lateral clavicle, spine of scapula and acromion.	Elevate and retract scapula. Assists in arm abduction by rotating the scapula.
Latissimus dorsi m.	SP of T_7 to L_3, thoracolumbar fascia, iliac crest, ribs 9–12 and inf. angle of scapula.	Bicipital groove.*	Extends, adducts, and medially rotates arm. Also, assists in deep inspiration and forceful expiration.
Levator scapulae m.	TP of C_1–C_4.	Medial border of scapula.	Raises medial scapula.
Teres major m.	Inf. angle of scapula.	Medial lip of bicipital groove.*	Medially rotates and adducts arm.
<u>T</u>eres minor m.†	From the upper ⅔ posterolateral border of scapula.	Lower facet of the greater tubercle of humerus.	Laterally rotates arm and weakly adducts it. Stabilizes glenohumeral joint.
<u>S</u>upraspinatus m.†	Medial border and spine of scapula (supraspinous fossa).	Greater tuberosity of humerus.	Abducts and stabilizes glenohumeral joint.
<u>I</u>nfraspinatus m.†	Medial border and spine of scapula (infraspinous fossa).	Greater tuberosity of humerus.	Laterally rotate and stabilizes glenohumeral joint.
<u>S</u>ubscapularis m.†	Medial subscapular fossa.	Lesser tuberosity of humerus.	Medially rotates arm and stabilizes glenohumeral joint.
Serratus anterior m.	Anterolateral surface of ribs 1–8.	Medial border of scapula.	Laterally rotates and protracts scapula.
Pectoralis major m.	Medial half of clavicle, lateral manubrium, sternum and costal cartilages of ribs 4–6.	Lateral lip of bicipital groove* and deltoid tuberosity.	Clavicular head: Flexes and adducts arm. Sternal head: Medially rotates and adducts arm.
Pectoralis minor m.	Anterior surface of ribs 3–5.	Coracoid process.	Elevates ribs with fixed scapula and protracts scapula.
Biceps brachii mm.	Long head: Supraglenoid tubercle of scapula. (Tendon passes through bicipital groove.) Short head: Coracoid process of scapula.	Bicipital aponeurosis and bicipital tubercle on proximal radius.	Primary supinator of forearm. Flexes elbow. They are also weak flexors of the shoulder.
Triceps Brachii mm.	Long head: Infraglenoid tubercle of scapula. Lateral head: Proximal ⅓ posterior humerus. Medial head: Mid-shaft posterior humerus.	Olecranon process of ulna.	The long head extends the glenohumeral joint. All three heads are recruited in forceful elbow extension.
Coracobrachialis m.	Coracoid process of scapula.	Medial mid-shaft of humerus.	Flexes and adducts (weak) arm.
Brachialis m.	Distal ⅔ of humerus.	Coronoid process of ulna.	Flexes elbow.
Pronator teres mm.	Humeral head: Medial epicondyle. Ulnar head: Coronoid process.	Lateral radius.	Pronates forearm and flexes elbow.

* All three mm. insert into the bicipital groove, from lateral to medial – Pectoralis **major** m., **Lati**ssimus dorsi m., and Teres **major** m.

 Memory Aid: **Lady** between **two majors.**

 Memory Aid: **SITS** mm. †These mm. form the rotator cuff.

The borders of which muscle divide the axillary artery into three parts?

The pectoralis minor m. divides the axillary a. into three parts (Figure 9.3).

 Memory Aid: The **first part** has **one branch**, the **second part** has **two branches**, and the **third part** has **three branches**.

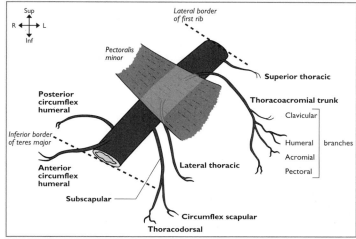

FIGURE 9.3 – Axillary artery.

The UE lymphatics ultimately drain into which group of axillary lymph nodes?

The apical lymph node group (Figure 9.4).

 Memory Aid: **APICAL** also serves as a mnemonic for all the groups of axillary lymph nodes—**A**pical, **P**osterior, **I**nfraclavicular, **C**entral, **A**nterior, and **L**ateral node groups.

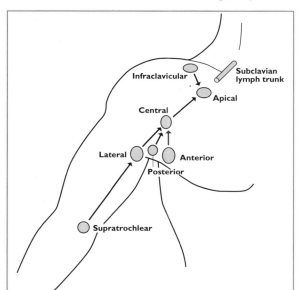

FIGURE 9.4 – Upper extremity lymphatics.

Shoulder Osteology (Figure 9.5)

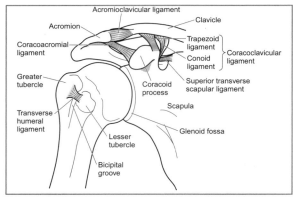

FIGURE 9.5 – Shoulder osteology.

Identify the labeled structures on the elbow radiograph (Figure 9.6):

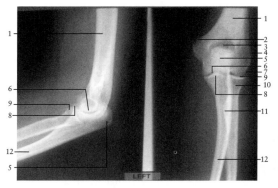

FIGURE 9.6 – Radiograph of the elbow (lateral and AP views).

1. Humerus
2. Medial condyle
3. Olecranon fossa
4. Lateral condyle
5. Olecranon process
6. Trochlea
7. Capitulum
8. Coronoid process
9. Radial head
10. Radial neck
11. Radial tuberosity
12. Ulna.

Which bone is the only connection between the shoulder and the axial skeleton?

The clavicle connects the scapula (at the acromion) to the manubrium of the sternum.

What structures can be found in the suprascapular notch?

1. Suprascapular **A**rtery (superiorly)
2. Superior transverse scapular ligament (middle)
3. Suprascapular **N**erve (inferiorly).

 Memory Aid: **A**rmy over **N**avy

What are the actions of the biceps brachii mm.?

Supination of the forearm > flexion of the elbow.

What nerve roots are responsible for the biceps clinical reflex? What about the triceps clinical reflex?

Biceps reflex: C5 nerve root.
Triceps reflex: C7 nerve root.

List the ligaments of the elbow.

1. Radial collateral ligament
2. Ulnar collateral ligament
3. Annular ligament

What is the carrying angle of the elbow?

The angle made when a longitudinal line through the humerus and a longitudinal line through the ulna intersect with complete elbow extension (in the anatomic position). Normal is 5 to 15 degrees.

Describe the interosseous membrane of the forearm.

It is a thickened fibrous sheath connecting the shafts of the radius and ulna that provides flexibility for pronation/supination motions. It also serves as an attachment for some forearm mm. and may transfer forces between the radius and ulna.

Identify the bones of the hand (Figure 9.7).

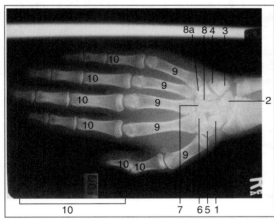

FIGURE 9.7 – Radiograph of the wrist and hand (AP view).

Proximal carpal row

1. **S**caphoid
2. **L**unate
3. **T**riquetrum
4. **P**isiform

Distal carpal row

5. **T**rapezium
6. **T**rapezoid
7. **C**apitate
8. **H**amate
   a. Hook of hamate

Hand

9. **M**etacarpals
10. **P**halanges

 Memory Aid: Carpal and Hand Bones
— **S**ome **L**ying **T**hieves
Play **T**ricks **T**hat **C**an
Hurt **M**any **P**eople.

What are the major components of the diaphragm of the wrist?

Carpal bones (proximal row), distal ends of radius and ulna, flexor and extensor mm. tendons, palmar and dorsal radioulnar ligaments, intercarpal ligaments, flexor retinaculum, and extensor retinaculum.

What structures can be found in the carpal tunnel?

The carpal tunnel formed by the distal row of carpal bones and flexor retinaculum contains the following (Figure 9.8):

1. Median n.

2. Flexor digitorum profundus tendons

3. Flexor digitorum superficialis tendons

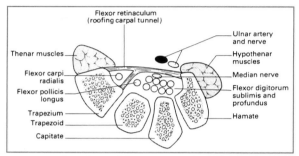

FIGURE 9.8 – Carpal tunnel (transverse section).

Where is the Tunnel of Guyon (Guyon's canal)?

It is found just lateral to the pisiform and the hook of hamate. The ulnar nerve and artery pass through this tunnel.

What is the anatomic "snuff box"? What are its contents?

A depression created on the dorsum of the hand with extension and abduction of the thumb. It is formed by the tendons of the abductor pollicis longus, extensor pollicis brevis, and extensor pollicis longus mm. The radial a., radial styloid process, scaphoid, and trapezium can all be palpated here.

How many dorsal interossei muscles are abductors?

Four **D**orsal interossei mm. **AB**duct the fingers.
Three **P**almar interossei mm. **AD**duct the fingers.

 Memory Aid: **4 DAB** and **3 PAD**

How do the actions of the flexor digitorum profundus m. and flexor digitorum superficialis m. differ?

Flexor digitorum profundus m. flexes the phalanges at the proximal interphalangeal (PIP) and distal interphalangeal (DIP) joint while the flexor digitorum superficialis m. flexes the middle phalanges at the PIP joints only.

CLINICAL ANATOMY

Identify the upper extremity neuropathies labeled in Figure 9.9. The answers are in Table 9.4.

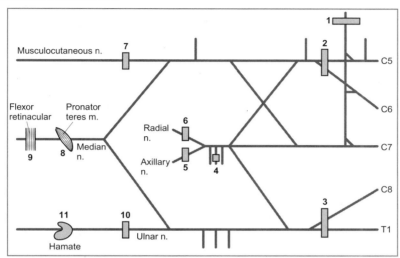

FIGURE 9.9 – Upper extremity neuropathies.

Name the nerve that can be injured with fractures of the following parts of the humerus.

Surgical neck	**Axillary n.**
Shaft (radial groove)	**Radial n.**
Distal humerus	**Median n.**
Medial epicondyle	**Ulnar n.**

What is the first long bone to begin ossification during development?	The clavicle. It is also the last bone to complete ossification and is the only long bone to undergo intermembranous ossification.
Where are clavicular fractures most common?	At the junction of the middle and lateral thirds ($\frac{1}{3}$ from the lateral end—weakest part of the clavicle).
How does a fractured clavicle appear on physical exam?	The medial $\frac{2}{3}$ will be elevated (due to sterno-cleidomastoid m.) while the lateral $\frac{1}{3}$ will be depressed (due to the weight of the upper limb) and pulled medially (due to pectoralis major m.).
What nerve injury will present with an inability to raise one's trunk/climb with the UE?	Thoracodorsal n., which innervates the latissimus dorsi m.

TABLE 9.4 – **Upper Extremity Neuropathies**

No.	Syndrome Name/ Nerve Injured	Presentation	Mechanism of Injury
1	Long thoracic n.	Posterolateral protrusion (winging) of the scapula	Axillary surgery or trauma
2	Erb (Duchenne) palsy Upper trunk	Waiter's tip	Fall on/trauma to shoulder and neck; complicated delivery (shoulder dystocia)
3	Klumpke's palsy Lower trunk	Claw hand	Hyperextension at shoulder with arm stretched above head
4	Thoracodorsal n.	Inability to raise one's trunk/climb with the upper extremity due to latissimus dorsi m. paralysis.	Axillary surgery or trauma
5	Axillary n.	Paralysis of deltoid/teres minor mm.	Surgical neck of humerus fractures
6	Saturday night palsy (crutch palsy) Radial n.	Wrist drop	Damage is a result of arm hanging over back of chair (drunk falls asleep), inappropriate crutch support, and fracture of humeral shaft through radial groove.
7	Musculocutaneous n.	Elbow flexion and forearm supination inability	Trauma to axilla
8	Pronator teres syndrome Median n.	Hand of benediction. Thenar wasting, hypoesthesia of first $3\frac{1}{2}$ digits, first 3 digits flexor weakness and wrist flexor weakness.	Spasm, hypertrophy, inflammation, fibrous bands or trauma to pronator teres m., bicipital aponeurosis or flexor digitorum superficialis m.
9	Carpal tunnel syndrome Median n.	Hand of benediction. Thenar wasting, paresthesia of first $3\frac{1}{2}$ digits, first 3 digits flexor weakness.	Processes that narrow the carpal tunnel such as inflammation, carpal bone dysfunction, edema/fluid retention (pregnancy and hypothyroid states), spasm, overuse, etc.
10	Ulnar n.	Claw hand (involves fourth and fifth digits only), hypoesthesia of last $1\frac{1}{2}$ digits, lateral blade of hand, hypothenar eminence, flexor carpi ulnaris m., and medial (ulnar) half of flexor digitorum profundus m.	Fractures and dislocations at the humeral medial epicondylar region.
11	Guyon's canal syndrome Ulnar n.	Claw hand (involves fourth and fifth digits only), hypoesthesia of last $1\frac{1}{2}$ digits, lateral blade of hand and hypothenar eminence.	Fracture of hamate, compression/ trauma to anteromedial wrist.

Injury to what nerve results in posterolateral protrusion of the scapula?	**Injury to the long thoracic n. (which innervates the serratus anterior m.) leads to medial rotation and posterior winging of the scapula. This winging is exaggerated by pushing anteriorly against a wall.** *Note: Trapezius m. paralysis (CN XI) can cause scapular winging and lateral rotation of the scapula.*
What is the most likely etiology of UE edema after a patient undergoes mastectomy?	In a radical and modified radical mastectomy, all the axillary lymph nodes deep to the pectoralis major m. are removed. These axillary lymph nodes drain the UE.
Anastomoses of what arteries allow for collateral circulation to the UE with axillary a. ligation?	Dorsal scapular a., suprascapular a., and subscapular a. (via the circumflex scapular a.) (See Figure 12.6C.)
What is the function of the rotator cuff?	In addition to the actions of the individual mm. (see Table 9.3), they collectively provide anterior, superior, and posterior stability to the glenohumeral (shoulder) joint.
Which is the most commonly injured tendon of the rotator cuff?	**Supraspinatus m. tendon**
What are the symptoms of a supraspinatus m. tendon tear?	The patient is unable to initiate active abduction at the shoulder or maintain abduction for prolonged periods (see arm drop test below). Tenderness may be found at the greater tubercle of the humerus.
What is a frozen shoulder?	A.K.A. adhesive capsulitis of the glenohumeral joint, results from fibrosis and inflammation of the joint capsule, shoulder bursa, rotator cuff mm., and/or deltoid m. Patient will have difficulty moving the shoulder, especially abducting the arm greater than 45 degrees. Commonly occurs in after shoulder/UE trauma where the patient immobilizes/guards the shoulder for an extended time.
Which is the most commonly dislocated major joint in the body?	The glenohumeral joint (a trade-off for its high range of motion).
What is the most common shoulder dislocation?	**Anterior shoulder dislocation. Abduction coupled with external rotation makes the anterior aspect of the joint capsule more vulnerable. (See apprehension test subsequently.)**
Crepitus and tenderness along the intertubercular (bicipital) groove of the humerus most likely represents ____.	Biceps tendonitis. This can result from repetitive microtrauma during athletic activities.

What is lateral epicondylitis (A.K.A. tennis elbow)?	**Inflammation and irritation of the lateral epicondyle, lateral collateral ligament (LCL), and extensor carpi radialis brevis m. This injury is a result of forceful extension of the wrist accompanied with a varus stress to the elbow, most commonly seen with the backhand stroke of tennis players.**
Describe medial epicondylitis (A.K.A. golfers elbow).	Inflammation and irritation of the medial epicondyle, medial collateral ligament (MCL), pronator teres, and wrist flexor mm. This injury is a result of forceful flexion of the wrist accompanied with a valgus stress to the elbow, most commonly seen with the swing of golfers.
Which vein is most commonly used for venipuncture?	Median cubital v. in the antecubital fossa.
What is nursemaid's elbow?	**The subluxation of the radial head due to excessive pull on a pronated forearm, commonly seen in children as they are pulled (by caretakers/ nursemaids). Severe cases can result in torn annular ligament.**
What nerve can be entrapped by the pronator teres m.?	**The median n. in pronator syndrome. Muscular spasm or hypertrophy, inflammation, fibrous bands, or trauma can lead to this syndrome.**
What is the most common fracture in adults over 50 years of age?	Fracture of the distal radius (more frequently in women due to osteoporosis).
Name and describe the most common fracture of the forearm.	Colle's fracture: complete transverse fracture with dorsal displacement of the distal radius from fall on an outstretched arm.
What are the presenting symptoms of carpal tunnel syndrome?	**Median nerve entrapment causes hypoesthesia/ paresthesia in the first three and a half digits. Patient may also have weakness and atrophy of the thenar mm.**
Which carpal bone is most commonly fractured?	Scaphoid fracture—this is the most common wrist injury as well.
Which carpal bone is most commonly dislocated?	The lunate bone most commonly dislocates anteriorly, often compressing the median n. (one of the causes of carpal tunnel syndrome).
What nerve is injured in a hamate fracture?	Ulnar nerve as it passes through the tunnel of Guyon.

What is Dupuytren's contracture?	**A fibrosis and contracture of the palmar aponeurosis. Patients present with painless nodular thickening and raised ridges over the palmar surface. Commonly seen in alcoholics.**
What is de Quervain's tenosynovitis?	A fibrosis, contracture, and stenosis of the tendinous sheaths of the abductor pollicis longus and extensor pollicis brevis mm. Wrist pain may radiate to forearm and thumb.
Describe a boxer's fracture.	Fracture of the neck of the fourth and fifth metacarpal bones.

Describe the following digital deformities and their associated disease processes.

Boutonniere's deformity	Extension at DIP and flexion at PIP (the shape of your finger when fastening a button). Seen with chronic rheumatoid arthritis (RA).
Swan neck deformity	Flexion at DIP and extension at PIP. Seen with chronic RA.
Ulnar deviation	Fingers sidebend medially at metacarpophalangeal toward ulna. Seen with chronic RA.
Bouchard's node	**Osteophytic (bony) overgrowth at the PIP joints forming enlarged nodular joints. Seen with RA.**
Heberden's node	**Osteophytic (bony) overgrowth at the DIP joints forming enlarged nodular joints. Seen with osteoarthritis.**
Trigger finger (digital tenovaginitis Stenosans)	Thickening of the fibrous digital sheath (palmar fibrous digital sheath) from overuse of fingers causing the inability to extend at the PIP/DIP joints.

OSTEOPATHIC PRINCIPLES

Which spinal segments supply autonomic innervation to the UE?	**Sympathetics: T1 or T2 to T8** **There is no parasympathetic supply to the extremities.**
How many articulations are involved in the shoulder joint?	True joints 1. Glenohumeral joint 2. Sternoclavicular joint 3. Acromioclavicular joint "Pseudo-joints" 4. Scapulothoracic "joint" 5. Suprahumeral "joint"

Describe the motions of the sternoclavicular joint and how it affects the UE.	A ball-and-socket type of joint that allows for clavicular movement and roll in the frontal and horizontal planes through an articular disc. Its anterior, posterior, superior, and inferior motions affect the motion of the upper extremity through the pectoral girdle. During complete upper limb elevation, the lateral end of the clavicle is raised 60 degrees.
What type of joint is the glenohumeral joint?	A ball-and-socket type of synovial joint, which allows for an extensive range of motion. Its relative instability and vulnerability to dislocation is often attributed to the wide range of motion (ROM).
What motions occur at the acromioclavicular joint?	1. Rotation of acromion on the clavicle 2. Minor gliding motion (accommodating for sternoclavicular movement)
Describe the two pseudo-joints of the shoulder	
Scapulothoracic "joint"	It is not a bony articulation; however, it functions as a joint due to the glide of the subscapularis m. on the serratus anterior m., a result of the combined sternoclavicular and acromioclavicular joints in motion. Elevation, depression, rotation, protraction, and retraction at this joint allow shoulder motion.
Suprahumeral "joint"	This joint is formed between the head of the humerus and the coraco-acromial ligament superiorly. This joint supports the motions of the glenohumeral joint and can potentially impinge several soft tissue structures (i.e., tendon of long head of biceps, supraspinatus, etc.).
Describe the following:	
Cubitus valgus	A carrying angle greater than 15 degrees.
Cubitus varus (gunstock deformity)	A carrying angle less than 5 degrees.
Describe the motions of the ulnohumeral joint type.	The ulnohumeral joint is a hinge-type of joint formed by the trochlear notch pivoting around the trochlea, which allows for flexion and extension at the elbow in one plane.
What motions occur at the radiohumeral joint?	The radiohumeral joint is a ball-and-socket joint allowing an axial rotation of the radius on the capitulum (supination/pronation of the forearm) and anterior/posterior glide (flexion/extension of elbow). The ball-and-socket joint would also allow for abduction/adduction; however, the accompanying ulnohumeral joint prevents this motion.

What motions are coupled with supination/pronation of the forearm?	<u>Sup</u>ination is coupled with <u>Add</u>uction of the elbow and anterior glide of the radial head. *Memory Aid:* <u>Add</u> <u>S</u>o<u>up</u>. <u>P</u>ronation is coupled with Abduction of the elbow and <u>p</u>osterior glide of the radial head. *Memory Aid:* <u>P</u>ronate for <u>P</u>osterior radial head.
What is the expected wrist dysfunction in persons with an adducted elbow (cubitus valgus)?	Ulnar deviation (adduction) at the wrist. Likewise, an abducted elbow (cubitus varus) will show radial deviation (abduction) at the wrist.

DIAGNOSIS

What constitutes a complete physical examination of the UE?	1. ROM at all major joints; compare passive and active bilaterally (see Table 9.1). 2. Radial head 3. Muscle tone and strength 4. Sensory function 5. Deep tendon reflexes 6. Vascular integrity (pulse) 7. Joint or dependent edema.
What findings should be noted when assessing joint motion and integrity?	Active/passive ROM, rigidity, crepitus, tenderness, inflammation, sensory deficit, and palpable nodularity.
Which major pulses are palpated to assess vascular integrity of the UE?	Brachial a., radial a., and ulnar a. *Remember: Perform the Allen test to assess hand perfusion; see subsequent section.*
How do you evaluate motion of the radial head?	Palpate the radial head on the lateral aspect of the elbow. Assess antero-posterior motion of the radial head by moving it back and forth.
What are the structural exam findings of an anterior radial head?	**The radial head is palpated in an anterior position; restriction in posterior glide will be present. Forearm supination freedom (pronation restriction) and adducted elbow are commonly found.**

What are the structural exam findings of a posterior radial head?	**The radial head is palpated in a posterior position; restriction in anterior glide will be present. Forearm pronation freedom (supination restriction) and abducted elbow are commonly found.**
Should the motion of the wrist and hand bones be assessed as group or as individual bones?	Individually.
What specific restrictions may be seen with the carpal and metacarpal bones?	Extension, flexion, ulnar deviation, radial deviation, and anterior/posterior glide.
How should carpal and metacarpal bone motion be tested?	Examiner palpates bone to be tested from the dorsal aspect, then locks out (immobilizes) adjacent bones with both thumbs dorsally while wrapping fingers around either side of the wrist/hand. Passive motion should then be tested.
How is the clinical diagnosis of "trigger finger" made?	Patient is unable to extend finger. When finger is extended passively, an audible snap is heard. Flexion also produces a snapping sound.

SPECIAL TESTS

Describe the following tests of the shoulder joint.

Adson's test or maneuver	**Patient seated while examiner finds and monitors radial pulse on arm being tested. Examiner passively abducts patient's arm to 90 degrees. Patient is asked to turn head toward shoulder being tested and extend their neck. Diminished or lost pulse may indicate thoracic inlet syndrome. Symptoms may be further exacerbated by deep inhalation.**

Apley scratch test

A general screening test for active range of motions of the shoulder joint. Elbow ROM may also be assessed with this test (Figure 9.10).

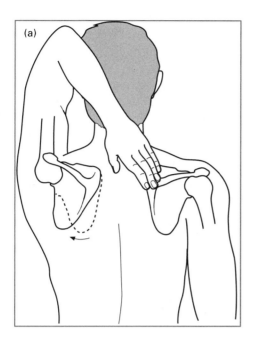

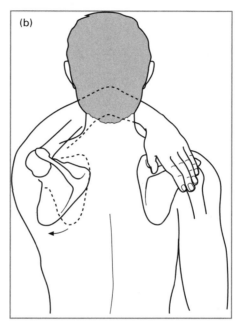

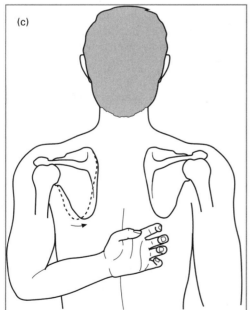

FIGURE 9.10 – Apley scratch test.

Apprehension test	**Examiner** places hand over anterior surface of patient's glenohumeral joint. **Examiner** then uses patient's forearm to externally rotate and abduct at the glenohumeral joint. Fear of dislocation (apprehension), active guarding, and pain indicate anterior glenohumeral instability (seen in patients with history of anterior shoulder dislocation).
Arm drop test	Patient seated or standing. **Examiner** abducts patient's arm to 90 degrees. **Examiner** taps on patient's arm. A positive sign is when the patient's arm drops quickly or severe pain accompanies action. This is useful for testing the rotator cuff (especially supraspinatus muscle/tendon).
Cross-flexion test	This tests for acromioclavicular ligament integrity. Patient's arm is abducted to 90 degrees and then adducted toward opposite shoulder (in front of chest wall). Gapping or pain at the acromioclavicular joint indicates a positive test result.
Trousseau's sign	Brachial a. occlusion (usually by a blood pressure cuff) can cause carpal spasm in hypocalcemic states.
Yerguson's test	**Examiner flexes patient's elbow to 90 degrees and monitors over the bicipital groove of the humerus. Using the patient's wrist, the shoulder is externally rotated. Patient is asked to internally rotate shoulder against resistance. Biceps long head tendon pain, clicking, or palpable movement (in and out of groove) indicates bicep tendon dislocation or tendonitis.**
What causes the diminished radial pulse in Adson's test?	Adson's maneuver causes the anterior scalene m. to raise the first rib, which narrows the thoracic inlet (compressing the subclavian artery).

Describe the following tests for the elbow joint:

Lateral epicondylitis test	**Patient is asked to make a fist. Examiner passively flexes wrist (thus, wrist and hand extensors are stretched). Patient is asked to extend wrist and/or digits against examiner's resistance. Pain, apprehension, or guarding indicates lateral epicondylitis.**
Medial epicondylitis test	**Patient is asked to make a fist. Examiner passively extends wrist (thus, wrist and hand flexors are stretched). Patient is asked to flex wrist and/or digits against examiner's resistance. Pain, apprehension, or guarding indicates medial epicondylitis.**

Valgus stress test	The patient's elbow is extended. While monitoring across the medial joint line, a force directed medially is applied to the lateral aspect of the elbow. Pain and gapping of the medial joint line are positive indicators of MCL injury.
Varus stress test	The patient's elbow is extended. While monitoring across the lateral joint line, a force directed laterally is applied to the medial aspect of the elbow. Pain and gapping of the lateral joint line are positive indicators of LCL injury.

Describe the following tests for the wrist and hand:

Allen's test	**Pressure is applied over the patient's radial and ulnar aa., occluding both of these vessels. The patient is asked to make a tight fist and release, repeating four to five times until the palm becomes pale. Examiner releases one of the vessels occluded and checks for reperfusion of the palm. The above is repeated testing for the other vessel. Reperfusion indicates patency of the vessel that was released.**
Finkelstein's test	Patient is asked to flex and adduct thumb and wrap fingers over thumb (making a fist). Then, patient is asked to adduct wrist (ulnar deviate). Pain or inability to ulnar deviate the wrist is a positive sign for de Quervain's tenosynovitis. This maneuver may make swelling or ganglion cysts more prominent as well.
Phalen's test	**Patient is asked to adduct arms at shoulder height, pushing dorsum of hands against each other (causing bilateral flexion of wrists). This may narrow the carpal tunnel resulting in symptoms of carpal tunnel syndrome.**
Tinel's sign	**Light tapping at the area of the flexor retinaculum may elicit symptoms similar to carpal tunnel syndrome (pain, paresthesia, etc.).**

TREATMENT

What treatment modalities are used in treatment of somatic dysfunctions of the UE?	All modalities may be used to treat the UE.
How can OMT decrease edema or vascular insufficiency?	Various lymphatic techniques of the UE (e.g., lymphatic effleurage, wobble technique, etc.) can improve venous and lymphatic return. Always remember to treat the thoracic inlet, pectoralis m. (overlies the axillary lymph nodes), and wrist diaphragms before treating the UE lymphatics.

113

What are common indications to perform the Spencer technique?	Adhesive capsulitis, first and second rib somatic dysfunction, thoracic inlet syndrome, and upper extremity edema. It can also be used in combination with muscle energy (ME) techniques for rotator cuff/shoulder m. strengthening and increasing shoulder ROM.
How is the Spencer technique performed?	Patient in lateral recumbent position with shoulder to be treated facing upward. Physician stabilizes scapula with one hand while other hand performs each of the following motions five to seven times (passively).
	1. Extension
	2. Flexion
	3. Circumduction with compression
	4. Circumduction with traction
	5. Abduction/Adduction
	6. Internal rotation
	7. Passive stretch
What osteopathic treatments are indicated in Nursemaid's elbow?	High velocity low amplitude (HVLA), muscle energy (ME), myofascial (MF), and counterstrain (CS) to the radial head.
List osteopathic techniques that may be used in treating Raynaud's phenomenon?	Treat autonomics to the UE, thoracic inlet, wrist diaphragm, and muscle/soft tissue impingements (which may decrease the blood flow to the hand).
Which modalities are particularly effective in treatment of UE tenosynovitis (de Quervain's, trigger finger, etc.)?	MF, ME, CS, and ligamentous articular strain (LAS) may be effective.
What are common contraindications to OMT of the UE?	1. Fracture
	2. Joint dislocation, infection, or open wound

GROSS ANATOMY OVERVIEW

Dermatomes of the Lower Extremity (Figure 10.1)

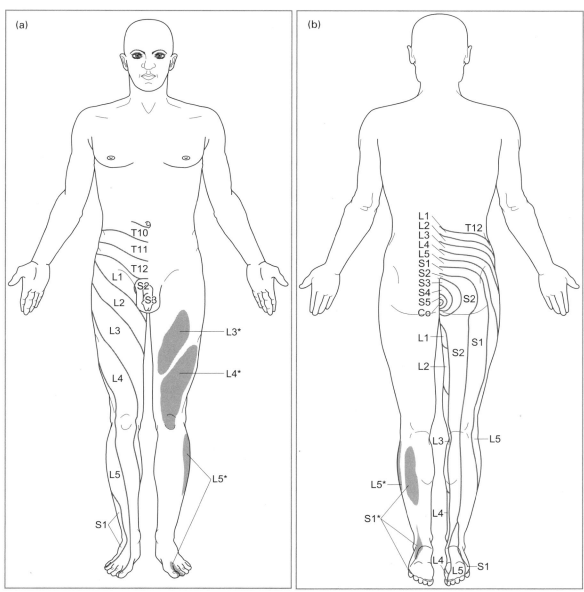

FIGURE 10.1 – Dermatomes of the lower extremity.

115

TABLE 10.1 – **Range of Motion of Lower Extremity Joints**

Joint	Motion	Range (in Degrees)
Hip	Flexion	0–120
	Extension	0–30
	Abduction	0–45
	Adduction	0–30
	External (lateral) rotation	0–45
	Internal (medial) rotation	0–45
Knee	Flexion	0–135
	Extension	0
Ankle	Flexion (plantarflexion)	0–50
	Extension (dorsiflexion)	0–20
	Inversion	0–35
	Eversion	0–15

Vasculature of the Lower Extremity (Figure 10.2)

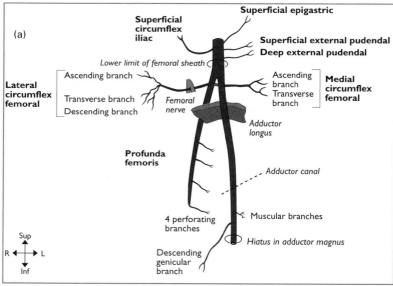

FIGURE 10.2 – Vasculature of the lower extremity. (a) Femoral artery; (b) popliteal artery; (c) anterior tibial artery; (d) posterior tibial artery; (e) peroneal (fibular) artery.

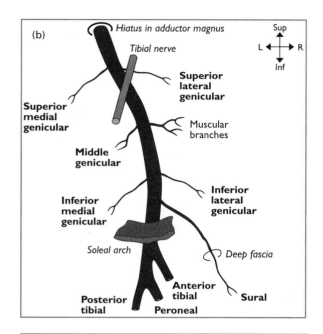

(b)

Hiatus in adductor magnus

Tibial nerve

Superior lateral genicular

Superior medial genicular

Muscular branches

Middle genicular

Inferior medial genicular

Inferior lateral genicular

Soleal arch

Deep fascia

Anterior tibial

Sural

Posterior tibial

Peroneal

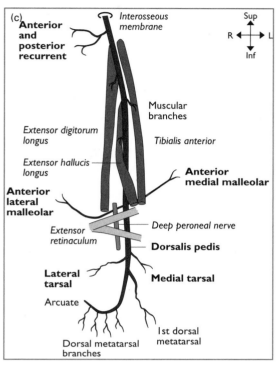

(c)

Anterior and posterior recurrent

Interosseous membrane

Muscular branches

Extensor digitorum longus

Tibialis anterior

Extensor hallucis longus

Anterior medial malleolar

Anterior lateral malleolar

Extensor retinaculum

Deep peroneal nerve

Dorsalis pedis

Lateral tarsal

Medial tarsal

Arcuate

1st dorsal metatarsal

Dorsal metatarsal branches

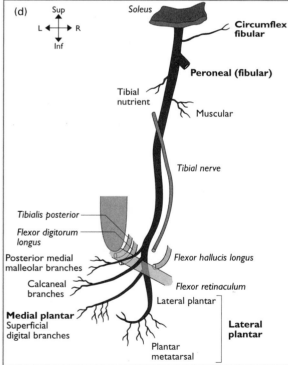

(d)

Soleus

Circumflex fibular

Peroneal (fibular)

Tibial nutrient

Muscular

Tibial nerve

Tibialis posterior

Flexor digitorum longus

Posterior medial malleolar branches

Flexor hallucis longus

Calcaneal branches

Flexor retinaculum

Lateral plantar

Medial plantar
Superficial digital branches

Lateral plantar

Plantar metatarsal

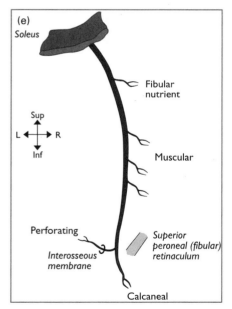

(e)

Soleus

Fibular nutrient

Muscular

Perforating

Superior peroneal (fibular) retinaculum

Interosseous membrane

Calcaneal

FIGURE 10.2 – *Continued*

The superficial inguinal lymph nodes drain lymph vessels from what structures?

Anterior abdominal wall (below umbilicus), perineum, urethra, external genitalia, and lower half of the anal canal.

Where do the superficial inguinal lymph nodes drain?

They drain into the deep inguinal lymph nodes then pass through the femoral canal and drain into the lymphatic system around the external iliac artery (Figure 10.3).

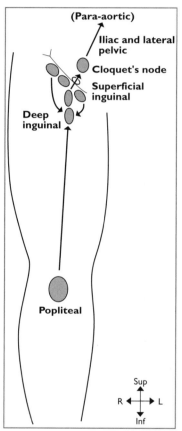

FIGURE 10.3 – Lower extremity lymphatics.

What type of joint is the hip?

Synovial ball and socket.

Osteology of the Femur (Figure 10.4)

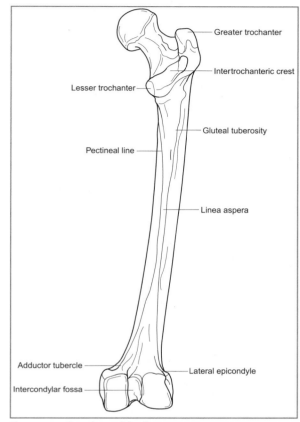

Greater trochanter

Intertrochanteric crest

Lesser trochanter

Gluteal tuberosity

Pectineal line

Linea aspera

Adductor tubercle

Lateral epicondyle

Intercondylar fossa

FIGURE 10.4 – Osteology of the femur.

What ligament connects the fovea to the acetabular fossa?	Ligamentum capitis femoris (A.K.A. ligament of femoral head or ligamentum teres). This ligament contains the acetabular branch of the obturator a., which supplies blood to the ligament (in children, it also supplies the femoral head).
Which artery is the main blood supply to the head of the femur in adults?	**Medial circumflex femoral a. from the profunda femoris a.**
The lunate surface of the acetabulum is continuous circumferentially except at __.	Acetabular notch (on the inferior portion of acetabulum). The transverse acetabular ligament lies over this notch.
Name the three major ligaments connecting the neck of the femur to the innominates.	1. **Ilio**femoral ligament 2. **Ischio**femoral ligament 3. **Pubo**femoral ligament *Memory Aid:* Think of the innominate bones—**ilio, ischio, and pubo**—attaching to the **femoral** neck.

119

Name the nerve that innervates the gluteus maximus muscle.	Inferior gluteal n. (L5–S2)
What muscle(s) is/are innervated by the superior gluteal n. (L4–S1)?	Gluteus medius, gluteus minimus, and tensor fasciae latae mm.
What structures pass through the greater sciatic foramen?	Superior and inferior gluteal nn./aa./vv., piriformis m., sciatic n., posterior femoral cutaneous n., pudendal n., internal pudendal a. and v., n. to quadratus femoris, and n. to obturator internus.
What structures pass through the lesser sciatic foramen?	**Pudendal n., internal pudendal a., obturator internus m.**

List the origins and insertions of the following muscles:

	Origin	Insertion
Iliopsoas m.	Vertebral bodies T_{12}–L_5, tranverse process of L_1–L_5, ilium and sacral ala	Lesser trochanter of femur
Piriformis m.	S_2–S_4 (ventral surface)	Greater trochanter
Gemellus superior m.	Spine of ischium	Greater trochanter
Gemellus inferior m.	Ischial tuberosity	Greater trochanter
Obturator internus m.	Obturator membrane and surrounding bone	Greater trochanter
Quadratus femoris m.	Ischial tuberosity	Intertrochanteric crest

What are the major muscles involved in hip flexion?	Iliopsoas (major flexor), sartorius, and rectus femoris mm.
What are the boundaries of the femoral triangle?	Lateral border: Sartorius m. Medial border: Adductor longus m. Superior border: Inguinal Ligament *Memory Aid:* The **SAIL** on a boat is **triangular**.

What structures are found in the femoral triangle?

From lateral to medial: Femoral <u>N</u>. → Femoral <u>A</u>. → Femoral <u>V</u>. → (<u>E</u>mpty space) → <u>L</u>ymphatics (Figure 10.5).

 Memory Aid: <u>**NAVEL**</u> going lateral to medial.

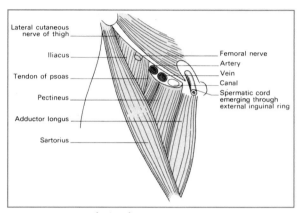

FIGURE 10.5 – Femoral triangle.

The superficial fascia of the thigh is continuous with what structure superiorly?

Superficial (Camper's) fascia of the abdominal wall.

What is the name of the opening through which the great saphenous vein drains into the femoral vein?

Saphenous opening.

What is the falciform margin?

The lower lateral border of the saphenous opening anterior to the femoral vessels.

What is the name given to the layer of membranous connective tissue that covers the saphenous opening?

Cribriform fascia.

Describe the course of the great saphenous vein and its function.

It drains a part of the dorsal venous arch of the foot, travels anterior to the medial malleolus, on the medial aspect of the leg, behind the knee, and finally drains into the femoral vein on the anteromedial aspect of the thigh. Throughout its course it has multiple connections to the small saphenous vein and communicates with deeper lower extremity veins via perforating branches (Figure 10.6).

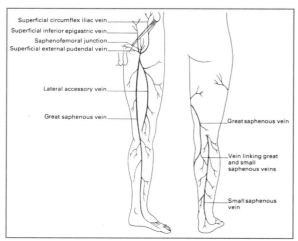

FIGURE 10.6 – Superficial veins of the leg.

List the muscles of each compartment of the thigh:

(Figure 10.7)

1. Anterior: sartorius, rectus femoris, vastus lateralis, vastus intermedius, vastus medialis, and iliopsoas mm.

2. Medial: gracilis, obturator externus, pectineus, adductor magnus, adductor longus, pectineus, and adductor brevis mm.

3. Posterior: long head of biceps femoris, short head of biceps femoris, semitendinosus, and semimembranosus mm.

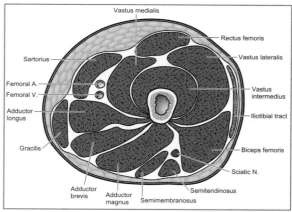

FIGURE 10.7 – Cross-section of the thigh.

What nerves can be found in each compartment of the thigh?

Anterior: femoral n. (L2–L4)

Medial: obturator n. (L2–L4)

Posterior: sciatic n. (L4–S3)

Describe the adductor hiatus (see Figure 10.2).

An opening in the distal portion of the adductor magnus m. that transmits the femoral vessels from the anterior thigh to the popliteal fossa posteriorly. The femoral vessels continue as popliteal vessels after they pass through.

Identify the labeled structures (Figure 10.8):

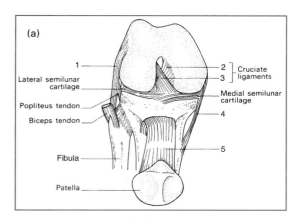

1. Lateral (fibular) collateral ligament
2. Posterior cruciate ligament (PCL)
3. Anterior cruciate ligament (ACL)
4. Medial (tibial) collateral ligament
5. Patellar ligament
6. Medial meniscus
7. Lateral meniscus.

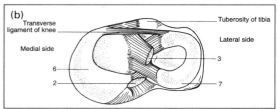

FIGURE 10.8 – Osteology of the knee. (a) Anterior view; (b) transverse section.

What bones make up the knee joint?

Femur, patella, and tibia—creating two articulations in the knee joint:

1. Patellofemoral
2. Tibiofemoral

What are the major components of the popliteal diaphragm?

Joint synovium and capsule, ACL, PCL, medial collateral ligament (MCL), lateral collateral ligament (LCL), transverse ligament of the knee, posterior meniscofemoral ligament, medial meniscus, lateral meniscus, popliteus m. and tendon, and articular surface of tibia and femur.

What is the term for the angle formed where a line connecting the anterior superior iliac spine to the middle of the patella meets a line connecting the tibial tubercle to the middle of the patella?

Q-angle, normally between 10 and 12 degrees.

What are the functions of the following knee structures:

ACL

ACL prevents excessive anterior slide of the tibia on the femur.

PCL

PCL prevents excessive posterior slide of the tibia on the femur.

LCL

Prevents excessive adduction of the leg at the knee.

MCL

Prevents excessive abduction of the leg at the knee.

The cruciate ligaments (anterior and posterior) of the knee are named for ___.

The location of their attachment to the tibia.

Identify the labeled structures (Figure 10.9):

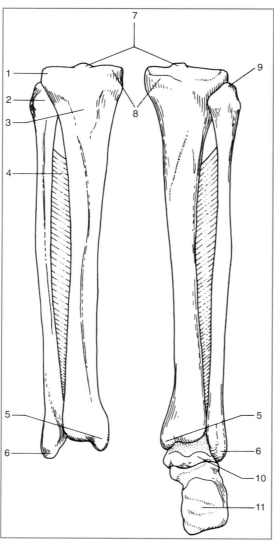

1. Lateral tibial condyle (plateau)
2. Fibular head
3. Tibial tuberosity
4. Interosseous membrane
5. Medial malleolus
6. Lateral malleolus
7. Intercondylar eminence
8. Medial tibial condyle (plateau)
9. Styloid process of fibula
10. Talus
11. Calcaneus

FIGURE 10.9 – Osteology of the leg.

What is the pes anserine?

The tendinous insertion point of the <u>S</u>artorius, <u>G</u>racilis, and Semi<u>T</u>endinosus mm. on the medial surface of the proximal tibia. Appears similar to a duck's foot. (French: *Pes* = foot, *Anserine* = duck)

 Memory Aid: Sergeant—**SGT.**

List the contents of each of the following compartments of the leg:

See Figure 10.10

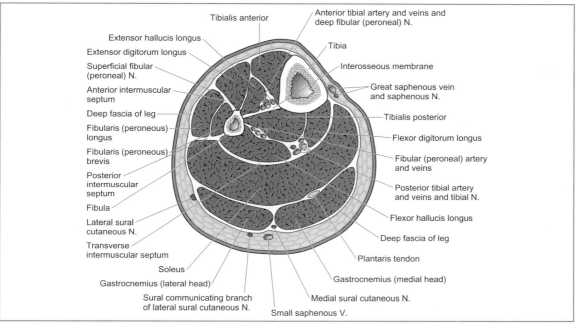

FIGURE 10.10 – Cross-section of leg.

Anterior compartment

Muscles: tibialis anterior m., extensor hallucis longus m., extensor digitorum longus m., fibularis (peroneus) tertius m.

Vessels: anterior tibial a. and v.

Nerves: deep fibular (peroneal) n.

Posterior compartment

Muscles: gastrocnemius (lateral and medial head) m., plantaris m., soleus m., popliteus m., flexor digitorum longus m., flexor hallucis longus m., tibialis posterior m.

Vessels: posterior tibial and fibular (peroneal) aa. and vv.

Nerves: tibial n. and superficial fibular (peroneal) n.

Lateral compartment

Muscles: fibularis (peroneus) longus m., fibularis (peroneus) brevis m.

Nerves: none (However, the muscles in this compartment are innervated by the superficial fibular n.)

125

What is the significance of the interosseous membrane?

It is a thickened fibrous sheath connecting the shafts of the tibia and fibula, dividing the anterior and posterior compartments. The interosseous membrane serves as an area of muscle origin and to transfer force between the tibia and fibula.

What structures can be found directly posterior to the medial malleolus?

From anterior to posterior: <u>T</u>ibialis posterior m. tendon → Flexor <u>D</u>igitorum longus m. tendon → Posterior Tibial <u>B</u>lood vessels → Tibial <u>N</u>. → Flexor <u>H</u>allucis longus m. tendon.

 Memory Aid: <u>T</u>om, <u>D</u>ick, and <u>B</u>loody <u>N</u>ervous <u>H</u>arry.

What are the major components of the diaphragm of the ankle?

Synovium & capsule, anterior talofibular (ATF) ligament, posterior talofibular ligament, calcaneofibular ligament, deltoid ligament, anterior tibiofibular ligament, posterior tibiofibular ligament, and posterior talocalcaneal ligament.

List the ligament(s) on the lateral aspect of the ankle joint.

1. ATF ligament
2. Posterior talofibular ligament
3. Calcaneofibular ligament.

Collectively they are known as the lateral ligament.

Name the ligament(s) on the medial aspect of the ankle joint.

Deltoid ligament (protects the ankle from eversion injuries).

Identify the labeled bones of the foot (Figure 10.11):

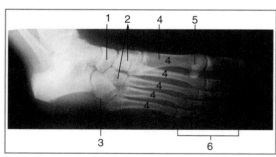

FIGURE 10.11 – Radiograph of foot.

1. Navicular
2. Cuneiforms (lateral, middle, and medial)
3. Cuboid
4. Metatarsals
5. Sesamoids
6. Phalanges

What are the natural arches of the foot?

1. Medial longitudinal arch
2. Lateral longitudinal arch
3. Transverse arches
   a. Anterior metatarsal transverse arch
   b. Posterior metatarsal transverse arch
   c. Tarsal transverse arch

Where is the spring ligament and what is its function?	Spring ligament (A.K.A. plantar calcaneonavicular ligament) runs from the sustentaculum tali to the navicular bone. Its major function is maintenance of the medial longitudinal arch of the foot.

CLINICAL ANATOMY

Describe Trendelenburg posture.	Standing with an externally rotated leg.

What nerve roots are evaluated in the following tests:

Knee Jerk (Patellar) deep tendon reflex (DTR)	L2, L3, L4
Ankle (Achilles) DTR	S1
Babinski (Plantar) Reflex	L4, L5, S1, S2 (up-going toe indicates upper motor neuron lesion—normal in infants up to 2 years age)
Heel Walk	L4, L5, S1, S2
Toe Walk	L4, L5, S1, S2, S3
Hallux Dorsiflexion (extension)	L5

Weakness in what hip muscle will result in difficulty to raise the trunk from a seated position?	**Gluteus maximus m.**
Where is the best location for intragluteal (intramuscular) injection? Why?	Superolateral quadrant to avoid damage to neurovascular structures found in other quadrants.
Spasm of what muscle will impinge on the sciatic nerve as it exits the greater sciatic foramen?	**The piriformis m. passes over the sciatic n. Piriformis m. spasm may lead to "piriformis syndrome."**
Localized inflammation traveling along the psoas major m. is indicative of what disease process?	Psoas abscess most commonly due to tuberculosis infection.
In order to catheterize the femoral vein, one must first palpate what structure?	Femoral arterial pulse, which lies directly lateral to the femoral v. in the femoral triangle.
What is a femoral hernia?	A protrusion of abdominal viscera through the femoral ring into the femoral canal (palpable in the femoral triangle).

Femoral hernias are more common in what gender?

Females. (But remember, the most common hernia in females is still an indirect inguinal hernia!)

 Memory Aid: **FEM**oral Hernia → **FEM**ale

In which position is the hip joint the least stable?

Adduction combined with internal rotation and flexion gives the hip the least stability. This position makes the hip most vulnerable to a posterior dislocation.

How does the angle of inclination for coxa vara and valga differ from the normal hip?

Coxa Vara—acute or ↓ angle of inclination
Coxa Valga—obtuse or ↑ angle of inclination
(Figure 10.12).

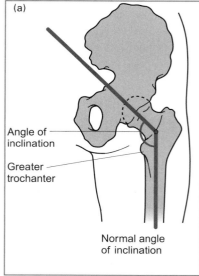
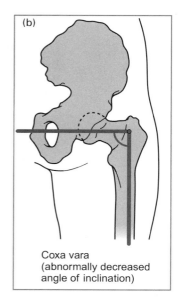
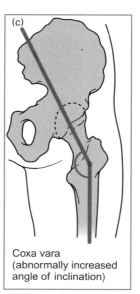

FIGURE 10.12 – Femoral angle of inclination.

What is the most common location of femoral fractures?

Anatomical neck

Femoral fractures are most common in what population?

Females older than 60 years (due to osteoporosis)

How does a patient with a femoral neck fracture present?

Fractured leg appears shortened and externally rotated (due to action of iliopsoas m.).

What vessels are vulnerable to injury with femoral neck fractures?

Medial circumflex femoral a. and lateral circumflex a.

Slipped capital femoral epiphysis (SCFE) is most common in what age group?	10 to 17 years of age.
What causes SCFE?	**A weakened epiphyseal plate resulting from acute trauma and repetitive microtrauma (obesity).**
What position makes a child more vulnerable to SCFE?	Abduction and lateral rotation.
What are the signs and symptoms of SCFE?	Hip discomfort and ↓ range of motion (ROM), referred knee pain, antalgic gait. Coxa vara tends to develop in these patients. *(See Figure 23.4 for radiograph of SCFE.)*
What causes avascular necrosis of the femoral head?	Compromise of the medial circumflex femoral a.
What are other names for Legg-Calvé-Perthes' disease?	Osteochondritis deformans juvenilis or aseptic necrosis of ossification center of femoral head.
What are the main signs and symptoms of Legg-Calvé-Perthes' disease?	**Pain from groin, hip, and thigh radiating to the knee with antalgic gait, ↑ ESR and psoas spasm.**
What is a "Charlie horse" (A.K.A. cricket thigh)?	Spasm or cramping of thigh mm. due to ischemia or contusion and rupture of blood vessels forming a hematoma.
Describe the following knee abnormalities:	
Genu Varum (Bow-legged)	Exaggerated medial angulation of the knee joint.
Genu Valgum (Knock-kneed)	Exaggerated lateral angulation of the knee joint.
What is the "unhappy triad" (A.K.A. O'Donaghue's triad) of knee injuries?	**<u>M</u>edial meniscus, <u>A</u>CL, and <u>M</u>CL injuries/sprains.** *Memory Aid:* Think <u>M</u> <u>A</u>nd <u>M</u>s playing football.
What is the mechanism of injury of the "unhappy triad"?	**Lateral clipping (valgus stress) with a rotation (twisting) on a fixed (planted) foot, most commonly from behind (as often seen in football injuries).**
How is the ACL most commonly damaged?	Sudden acceleration-deceleration and twisting mechanisms.

What is the most common mechanism of PCL injury?	Posterior displacement of the proximal tibia with a flexed knee (as seen with knees hitting dashboards in automobile collisions).
What injuries can be expected with a:	
Varus stress?	LCL
Valgus stress?	MCL accompanied with possible medial meniscal tear.
Why is a medial meniscal tear commonly found with an MCL tear?	Fibers from the MCL insert into the medial meniscus, thus injury to the MCL can lead to injury of the medial meniscus. The LCL does not insert on the lateral meniscus.
Where is a "Baker's cyst" located?	**Popliteal fossa. It is an out-pocketing of the knee synovium, commonly associated with rheumatoid arthritis.**
What is "housemaid's knee"?	Chronic bursitis of the knee resulting in inflammation and edema in the infrapatellar region. *Memory Aid:* Think of a housemaid down on her knees scrubbing the floor
Point tenderness and inflammation at the tibial tubercle is a common finding in what disease?	Osgood-Schlatter disease. The pain is caused by traction and relieved with rest.
What causes varicose veins?	Dilation of the great saphenous v. (and its tributaries) to the point of venous valvular insufficiency.
What is the likely cause of unilateral lower extremity edema status-post coronary artery bypass graft (CABG)?	**Decreased venous return from the LE due to removal of the great saphenous v. for the CABG.**
What causes compartment syndrome?	Trauma or burn to leg muscles can result in hemorrhage, edema, and inflammation in the leg compartments. This can cause an increase in intra-compartment pressure great enough to compress adjacent structures (vessels and nerves) (see Figures 10.7 and 10.10).
What are signs and symptoms of compartment syndrome?	**Decreased motor function in muscles of an individual compartment and decreased temperature distal to the compression. All of these may not be present simultaneously in a compartment syndrome. Vessel compression may occur; however, loss of distal pulses is a very rare and severe finding.**

What causes the pain and edema in the distal two-thirds of the tibia in "shin splints" (anterior tibialis strain)?	Repetitive microtrauma to the tibial periosteum and tibialis anterior m. This can be considered a mild form of "anterior compartment syndrome." It is commonly seen in sedentary individuals who attempt to participate in physically strenuous exercises without training or stretching (i.e., marathons).
List the signs and symptoms of common fibular (peroneal) n. injury.	Loss of eversion, dorsiflexion (foot drop), and sensation to the anterolateral leg and dorsum of foot. They will compensate by a high stepping gait (steppage).
Inability to plantarflex indicates injury to what nerve?	Tibial n. (L4–S3)
What is the most commonly injured major joint?	Ankle; especially sprains.
What is the most common mechanism of ankle sprain?	Inversion accompanied with hyperflexion (plantarflexion).
Which is the most commonly injured ligament of the ankle?	**A**nterior **T**alo**F**ibular ligament. 🐍 *Memory Aid:* **ATF**—**A**lways **T**ears **F**irst **The calcaneofibular ligament is the second most commonly torn.**
Name the fracture that may occur during forceful foot eversion and dislocation of the ankle.	Pott's fracture of the medial malleolus.
Where can the dorsalis pedis a. pulse be palpated?	Lateral to the extensor hallucis longus tendon. (Tendon is exaggerated with extension/dorsiflexion of the ankle and great toe.)
What is a fracture at the base of the fifth metatarsal known as?	**Jones' fracture (occurs through the metatarsal diaphysis).**
What muscle is affected in an avulsion fracture of the fifth metatarsal tuberosity?	**Fibularis brevis m. This avulsion fracture is also known as a pseudo-Jones' fracture.**
How does a plantar fasciitis typically present?	Generally no pain at rest, severe heel pain with weight bearing and after being seated for long periods. Pain improves gradually with activity. Straining and inflammation of the plantar aponeurosis can be noted at its origin on the medial tubercle of the calcaneus. Typically, a marathon runner with worn out shoes complaining of heel pain.

What is a "heel spur"?	Protrusion of an abnormal bony process from the medial calcaneal tubercle that often becomes inflamed and painful.

Describe the following foot deformities:

Pes planus (Flat foot)	Longitudinal arches are flattened.
Pes equinus	Plantarflexed ankle causing toe walk.
Pes calcaneus	Dorsiflexed ankle causing heel walk.
Talipes equinovarus (Clubfoot)	Pes equinus superimposed with inversion, forefoot adduction, and calcaneal varus due to shortened gastrocnemius.
Morton's syndrome	Shortened first metartarsal. Patient may present with great toe shorter than second digit accompanied by pain.
Morton's neuroma	Fibroneuromatous reaction between distal ends of metatarsals, commonly third and fourth.
Claw toe	Hyperextension of the metatarsal phalangeal (MTP) with flexion of distal interphalangeals (DIPs).
Hammer toe	Hyperextension of the MTP and DIP with a flexed proximal interphalangeal.
Hallux valgus	Abduction (lateral deviation) of the great toe (crossing over second digit).
Bunion	Inflammation and pain localized to a plantar bursa from friction.
Callus	Pressure reaction leading to hyperkeratosis.
Soft corns	Hyperkeratosis between toes, commonly fourth or fifth toes.
Hard corns	Inflamed areas of thick skin over hyperflexed or hyperextended joints.

Describe the two phases of gait cycle.

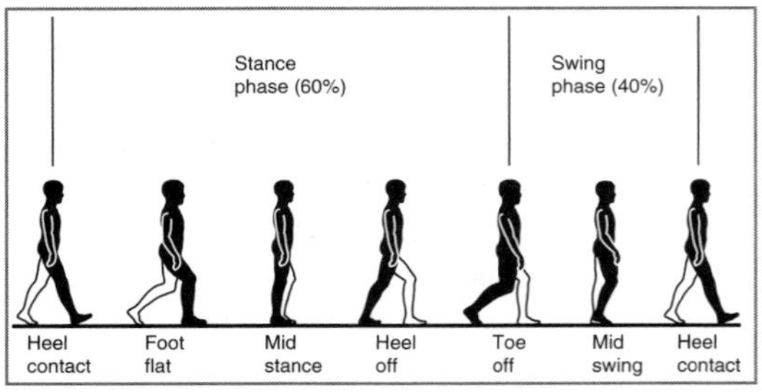

Stance Phase

1. Heel strike
2. Foot flat
3. Mid-stance
4. Heel-off
5. Toe-off

Swing Phase

1. Toe-off
2. Mid-swing
3. Heel strike

(Figure 10.13)

FIGURE 10.13 – Phases of gait.

How does the gait of patients with injury or paralysis of the following muscles present:

Gluteus maximus or hamstring mm.	Lean backward during heel-strike.
Vasti mm.	Lean forward during heel-strike.
Iliopsoas	Unable to walk.
Adductor mm.	Flexion during early swing phase accompanied by some abduction.
Anterior compartment of leg mm.	High-stepping gait (similar to common peroneal n. injury above).

Describe Trendelenburg gait.	Seen in patients with injured superior gluteal n. (commonly secondary to poliomyelitis). This results in weakness of the gluteus medius and minimus mm. as well as the tensor fasciae latae m. During the stance phase of the affected leg, the opposite hip drops (see Trendelenburg test below) and the patient side bends toward the affected leg to compensate.

OSTEOPATHIC PRINCIPLES

Which spinal segments supply autonomic innervation to the lower extremity (LE)?	**Sympathetics: T10 or T11–L2.** **There is no parasympathetic supply to the extremities.**
What are the advantages of the ball-and-socket joint at the hip?	It allows for motion in all three planes along with circumduction.
List the functions of the tensor fasciae latae muscle.	Assists in keeping the knee in extension while exerting traction on the iliotibial tract. It also acts as a hip abductor in conjunction with the lesser gluteal mm. during gait.
List the main muscles of hip extension.	Gluteus maximus, lateral hamstring (long and short head of biceps femoris) and medial hamstring (semimembranosus and semitendinosus) mm.
Name the major abductors of the hip.	Gluteus medius, gluteus minimus, tensor fasciae latae, sartorius mm. (the piriformis m. also causes abduction when the hip is in a flexed position).
What hip muscles are major adductors?	Adductor magnus, adductor longus, adductor brevis, gracilis, pectineus mm.

List the major medial (internal) rotators of the hip joint.	**Gluteus medius**, gluteus minimus, tensor fasciae latae, adductor mm.
Which muscles laterally (externally) rotate the thigh at the hip joint?	**Piriformis**, gluteus maximus, gemellus superior, gemellus inferior, obturator internus, obturator externus, quadratus femoris mm.
What is the function of the patella in knee extension?	The patella serves as a pulley for the distal LE by using the contraction force of the quadriceps muscles to extend the knee joint via the patellar ligament.
How does the sellar-type patellofemoral joint assist in knee extension?	The sellar-type joint allows longitudinal glide of the patella within the intercondylar groove (of the femur) as the extensor muscles contract and relax.
What are the primary actions of the quadriceps femoris mm.?	Extension of the knee > Flexion of the hip.
What muscle is the most powerful extensor of the knee?	**Vastus lateralis m. This muscle is so powerful that it can cause the patella to track laterally, especially in females due to their wider hips.**
Motion at which joint is coupled with fibular head motion?	Ankle joint.
How do the motions of the two ends of the fibula relate to each other?	Anterior and posterior movement of the distal fibula results in the opposite motion of the fibular head. This is due to the fulcrum-like action of the interosseous membrane.
What motions of the ankle are coupled with the fibular head? Why?	1. **Dorsiflexion, abduction, external rotation, and eversion of the ankle cause posterior movement of the distal fibula → anterior glide of the fibular head.** 2. **Plantarflexion, adduction, internal rotation, and inversion of the ankle cause anterior movement of the distal fibula → posterior glide of the fibular head.**
Describe pronation of the foot.	**A-B-duction, dorsiflexion (Extension), and Eversion of the ankle during Pronation.** (image) ***Memory Aid:* BEEP.**
What ankle motions comprise supination of the foot?	**A-D-duction, Inversion, and Plantarflexion during Supination.** (image) ***Memory Aid:* DIP** in **S**oup.

What are the functions of the plantar arches?	Shock absorption and resistance to excessive ankle dorsiflexion during gait.
In which plantar arch are somatic dysfunctions most common?	Transverse arch.
Which bones of the foot are affected by somatic dysfunction of the (tarsal) transverse arch?	The second cuneiform, the medial edge of the cuboid, and the lateral edge of the navicular all glide inferiorly.
Which of the arches is the largest and why?	The medial longitudinal arch has the greatest height, length, and width. This is due to the great forces across this arch generated by the plantar ligaments, tibialis posterior m., flexor digitorum longus m., and intrinsic muscles of the foot.
How can flattening of the plantar arches result in dysfunctions elsewhere in the body?	Flattening of the plantar arches can lead to inferior displacement of the major body joints above the foot (leading to sacral base unleveling and other compensatory patterns throughout the body).

DIAGNOSIS

What assessments should be made when observing a patient's gait?	1. Symmetry of legs 2. Weight bearing on both legs 3. Body position (forward, backward or sidebending) 4. Time in each phase of gait 5. Length of each step 6. Use of support (e.g., cane, walker, crutches, wall, etc.) 7. Balance 8. Speed 9. Exertion 10. Active ROM at all joints 11. Foot clearance
What constitutes a complete physical examination of the LE?	1. ROM at all major joints, compare passive and active bilaterally (see Table 10.1). 2. Fibular head and talotibial joint motion 3. Plantar arches 4. Muscle tone and strength 5. Sensory function 6. DTRs 7. Vascular integrity (pulse) 8. Joint or dependent edema 9. Gait

How do you evaluate motion of the fibular head?	Palpate the fibular head on the lateral aspect of the leg. Assess anteroposterior motion of the fibular head by moving it back and forth.
What are the physical exam findings of an anterior fibular head?	Resistance to posterior spring, distal fibula palpated posteriorly, and/or eversion and dorsiflexion (due to external rotation of talus).
What are the physical exam findings of a posterior fibular head?	Resistance to anterior spring, distal fibula palpated anteriorly, and/or inversion and plantarflexion (due to external rotation of talus).
How do you evaluate motion at the talotibial joint?	With the hip and knee extended, check plantar and dorsiflexion at the ankle joint. An anterior tibia will restrict dorsiflexion, whereas an anterior talus will restrict plantarflexion.
Name and describe the dysfunctions of the talotibial joint.	1. Anterior tibia on talus: presents with restricted dorsiflexion. 2. Anterior talus on tibia: presents with restricted plantarflexion (because posteriorly displaced tibia will prevent this motion).
Should the motion of the foot bones be assessed as group or as individual bones?	Individually.
What specific restrictions may be seen with the calcaneus bone?	Restriction in eversion and inversion.
What restrictions do the cuboid and navicular bones exhibit?	Dorsal glide restriction or plantar (ventral) glide restriction.
What types of motions should the metatarsals and the cuneiforms be checked for?	Dorsal-ventral translation and internal-external rotation.
Which major pulses are palpated to assess vascular integrity of the LE?	1. **Femoral a. pulse** 2. **Popliteal a. pulse** 3. **Posterior tibial a. pulse** 4. **Dorsalis pedis a. pulse** **Besides palpating the above pulses, you may also assess warmth, hair growth, and capillary refill of the LE/foot.**
How is the medial plantar arch evaluated?	Barefoot patient stands erect with feet shoulder-width apart. Examiner slides fingertips under medial plantar arches bilaterally. There will be less clearance for fingertips with flattened medial plantar arches.

How is leg length evaluated clinically?

Patient is supine. Patient is asked to place feet flat on table, bend knees, and raise hips to square position. Patient returns to supine position with hips and knees extended. Positions of the medial malleoli are compared to assess length of the legs. To neutralize for positional asymmetry, perform the FAbERE motion (see subsequent section, Special Tests) and reassess.

SPECIAL TESTS

Describe the following tests for the hip and their significance.

Thomas' test

Patient supine and flexes both hips and knees to level of chest. Patient then extends one leg while holding other knee to chest. In cases of iliopsoas m. spasm, patient will be unable to completely extend hip and knee in affected extremity. Patient may also increase lumbar lordosis in a positive test result.

Ober's test

Patient lies on unaffected side. Examiner abducts top leg and releases it. In cases of ilio-tibial band contracture, the affected (top) leg will not drop freely.

Ortolani's test

Baby is supine; examiner flexes hip and knees with index fingers on the greater trochanter and thumbs over the lesser trochanter bilaterally. Simultaneously abduct, externally rotate, then extend the legs. In cases of congenitally dislocated hip, the examiner may feel or see a "clunk" or hear a "click."

FAbERE's (Patrick's) test

Patient is supine; their hip is Flexed, Abducted, Externally Rotated, and then Extended (thus the name F-Ab-ER-E). It is primarily a ROM test, but may also be used to screen for crepitus and degenerative joint disease (DJD) of the hip. This test may also be used to test the sacroiliac joint.

Trendelenburg test

Standing patient is asked to raise one leg while shifting body weight to opposite leg. With normal gluteal strength, iliac crest on side of raised leg should also rise or remain level. In cases of gluteus medius weakness of the stance leg, the contralateral (the side the leg is raised) iliac crest will drop lower when same leg is raised.

Ludloff's sign

Ecchymosis in the femoral triangle indicates traumatic epiphyseal separation of the lesser trochanter.

Straight leg raise	With patient supine, raise and extend one leg slowly. Patient complaints of lower back pain or radiating leg pain may indicate lumbar disc herniation or sciatic nerve impingement.
Galezzi's sign	In cases of congenital hip dislocation or dysplasia, the thigh/leg may appear shorter.

Describe the following tests for the knee and their significance.

Valgus stress test	The knee is flexed 5 degrees. While monitoring across the medial joint line, a force directed medially is applied to the lateral aspect of the knee. Pain and gapping of the medial joint line are positive indicators of MCL injury.
Varus stress test	The knee is flexed 5 degrees. While monitoring across the lateral joint line, a force directed laterally is applied to the medial aspect of the knee. Pain and gapping of the lateral joint line are positive indicators of LCL injury.
Anterior draw test	Patient supine with knee flexed 90 degrees. Examiner stabilizes foot while placing thumbs over the tibial tuberosity and wrapping fingers around proximal tibia. The examiner directs an anterior force on the proximal tibia. Excessive anterior gliding of the tibia indicates a positive test result.
Posterior draw test	Patient supine with knee flexed 90 degrees. Examiner stabilizes foot while placing thumbs over the tibial tuberosity and wrapping fingers around proximal tibia. The examiner directs a posterior force on the proximal tibia. Excessive posterior gliding of the tibia indicates a positive test result.
Lachman's test	Patient supine with knee flexed 20 to 25 degrees. Examiner places one hand behind proximal tibia and other hand on top of distal thigh. A force is applied, drawing the tibia anteriorly while stabilizing the thigh. Excessive anterior gliding of the tibia indicates a positive test result.
McMurray's test	Patient is supine. There are four steps to the test:

1. Examiner flexes hip and knee. While internally rotating at the knee and applying a valgus stress to the knee, the hip and knee are extended.
2. Examiner flexes hip and knee. While externally rotating at the knee and applying a valgus stress to the knee, the hip and knee are extended.
3. Examiner flexes hip and knee. While internally rotating at the knee and applying a varus stress to the knee, the hip and knee are extended.

4. Examiner flexes hip and knee. While externally rotating at the knee and applying a varus stress to the knee, the hip and knee are extended.

Pain indicates a positive sign that implies meniscal damage. Steps 1 and 2 (valgus stress) test for lateral meniscus and steps 3 and 4 (varus stress) test for medial meniscus.

Apley's compression test

Patient is prone while examiner stabilizes distal thigh. Patient's knee is flexed to 90 degrees and a downward/compressing force is applied through the foot toward the knee. Pain indicates a positive sign that implies meniscal damage.

Apley's distraction test

Patient is prone while examiner stabilizes distal thigh. Patient's knee is flexed to 90 degrees and an upward/distracting force is applied to the knee using the foot. Pain indicates a positive sign that implies ligamentous injury.

Patellofemoral grinding

Patient's knee is extended and leg muscles are relaxed. A downward force is applied through the center of the patella on the femur while simultaneously gliding patella over femur. Pain and crepitus are positive signs indicating DJD.

Bounce home test

Patient is supine while examiner completely flexes the knee, supporting LE from the heel. The examiner allows the knee to fall into extension freely. Normal patients will come to an abrupt and complete stop at full extension. Laxity in the end-point of extension indicates a meniscal tear.

Patellar apprehension test

Patient is supine with leg muscles relaxed. Examiner flexes knee to 30 degrees while distracting the patella laterally. If patient reports patellar dislocation or exhibits knee guarding, it is a positive test result. A positive test result is indicative of a history of patellar dislocation.

Patellar translation

Patient is supine with leg muscles relaxed. Examiner translates/glides patella over femur supero-inferiorly and mediolaterally while checking for crepitus, lateral tracking, and pain. This test can be diagnostic of DJD or patellofemoral syndrome.

Describe the following tests for the ankle and their significance.

Thompson's test

Patient is prone, examiner flexes knee and squeezes calf muscles. Intact Achilles tendon will cause plantar flexion. Pain or lack of plantar flexion indicates an Achilles tendon injury.

Anterior draw sign	Examiner stabilizes LE proximal to ankle with one hand while cupping the heel with the other. The ankle joint is held at 20 degrees dorsiflexion. Examiner distracts foot anteriorly (by the heel). Increased anterior mobility represents weakness of the ATF ligament, anterior joint capsule, and/or calcaneofibular ligament.
Homan's sign	**Patient is supine, examiner dorsiflexes foot. Pain in the calves indicates a positive test result, which indicates possible deep venous thrombosis.**
Valgus stress test	A force directed medially is applied to the lateral aspect of the ankle (causing eversion) while monitoring across the medial joint line. Pain and gapping of the medial joint line are positive indicators of deltoid ligament injury.
Varus stress test	A force directed laterally is applied to the medial aspect of the ankle (causing inversion) while monitoring across the lateral joint line. Pain and gapping of the lateral joint line are positive indicators of calcaneofibular ligament injury.

TREATMENT

What treatment modalities are used in treatment of somatic dysfunctions of the LE?	All modalities may be used to treat the LE.
What is the osteopathic treatment for piriformis syndrome?	Counterstrain (CS), facilitated positional release, myofascial (MF), muscle energy to piriformis m. Correct hip, sacral, and innominate dysfunctions.
What is sacral base unleveling (SBU)?	Sacral base asymmetry due to sidebending of the sacrum along an anteroposterior axis as a result of leg length discrepancies. It is most commonly assessed using radiographic studies. SBU > $\frac{1}{8}$–$\frac{1}{4}$ inch requires lift therapy.
How is the amount of lift required for treatment of anatomic short leg syndrome determined?	Lift required = SBU/(D + C) Duration (D) is graded on a scale of 1 to 3:

1 = 1 to 10 years

2 = 11 to 30 years

3 = greater than 30 years

Compensation (C) is graded on a scale of 0 to 2:

0 = Sidebending only

1 = Sidebending with rotation in opposite directions

2 = Anatomical changes such as wedging and facet degeneration

How can OMT decrease edema or vascular insufficiency?

Various lymphatic techniques of the LE (e.g., pedal pump, wobble technique, etc.) can improve venous and lymphatic return. Always remember to treat the abdominal, pelvic, popliteal, and ankle diaphragms before treating the LE lymphatics.

List the contraindications to pedal pump.

Absolute contraindication

- **Venous thrombus**

Relative contraindications

- **LE injury**

Congestive heart failure
Cellulitis, local infection, or abscess

How can treatment of muscle spasm or inflammation improve compromised blood flow or nervous function?

Relief from spasms and inflammation help to decrease the tension that muscles can place on neurovascular structures within their respective compartments (as in compartment syndrome).

Which modalities are particularly effective in treatment of plantar fasciitis?

MF, CS, ligamentous articular strain, and lymphatic effleurage.

SECTION IV

Cranial Anatomy and Osteopathy

11 CRANIUM

GROSS ANATOMY OVERVIEW

Name all the paired bones of the adult neurocranium.	**Parietal and temporal bones.** *Note: In craniosacral motion, the frontal bone acts as a paired bone.*
Name all the unpaired bones of the facial skeleton (viscerocranium).	**Mandible and vomer.**

Identify the following structures (Figure 11.1):

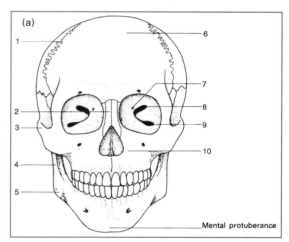

1. Coronal suture
2. Nasal bone
3. Zygomatic arch
4. Ramus of mandible
5. Angle of mandible
6. Frontal bone
7. Optic foramen
8. Superior orbital fissure
9. Inferior orbital fissure
10. Maxilla
11. Hard palate
12. Lateral pterygoid plate
13. External auditory meatus
14. Mastoid process
15. Foramen magnum
16. Occipital bone
17. Medial pterygoid plate
18. Carotid canal
19. Styloid process
20. Stylomastoid foramen
21. Jugular foramen
22. Occipital condyle.

FIGURE 11.1 – Cranial osteology (a and b).

TABLE II.I – **Cranial Foramina**

Foramen	Structure(s) Passing Through
Foramina of cribriform plate	CN I nerve bundle
Optic canal	CN II and ophthalmic artery
Superior orbital fissure	CN III, CN IV, CN V_1 (ophthalmic n.), CN VI, superior ophthalmic v.
Foramen rotundum	CN V_2 (Maxillary n.)
Foramen ovale	CN V_3 (Mandibular n.)
Foramen spinosum	Middle meningeal vessels
Carotid canal	Internal carotid artery and nerve plexus
Internal acoustic meatus	CN VII and CN VIII
Jugular foramen	CN IX, CN X, CN XI and sigmoid sinus → internal jugular v.
Hypoglossal canal	CN XII
Foramen magnum	Medulla oblongata, meninges, vertebral aa., and spinal roots of accessory n.

What is the name for the H-shaped congregation of the sutures located at the junction of the frontal, parietal, sphenoid (greater wing), and temporal bones?

Pterion.

Describe the asterion.

A *star*-shaped landmark located at the junction of the parietomastoid, occipitomastoid, and lambdoid sutures. This is the region where the parietal, temporal, and occipital bones meet.

 Memory Aid: **Asteroids** are in the sky with **stars**.

What is the most prominent posterior point of the external occipital protuberance?

The inion.

What are the layers of the scalp?

Skin, **C**onnective tissue, **A**poneurosis (epicranius m.), **L**oose connective tissue, and **P**ericranium.

 Memory Aid: **S C A L P**.

Identify the following structures (Figure 11.2):

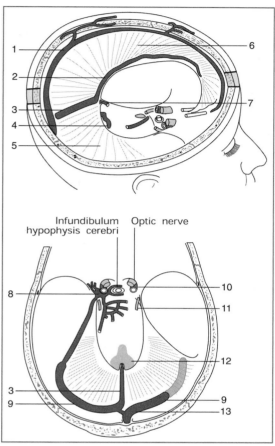

FIGURE II.2 – Venous sinuses and dura.

1. Superior sagittal sinus
2. Inferior sagittal sinus
3. Straight sinus
4. Sigmoid sinus
5. Tentorium cerebelli
6. Falx cerebri
7. Great cerebral vein
8. Cavernous sinus
9. Transverse sinus
10. Internal carotid a.
11. Oculomotor n. (CN III)
12. Foramen magnum
13. Confluence of sinuses.

What are the three layers of the cranial meninges?	1. Dura mater: thick outer meningeal fibrous tissue 2. Arachnoid mater: thin middle meningeal membrane 3. Pia mater: inner vascular meningeal membrane.
How do dural in-foldings (reflections) separate different regions of the brain?	The external periosteal layer of dura separates from the internal meningeal layer creating the in-foldings referred to as the falx cerebri, tentorium cerebelli, falx cerebelli, and diaphragma sellae (see Figure 11.2).
Which dural layer secretes cerebrospinal fluid (CSF)?	The choroid plexuses are highly vascular fringes of pia mater that secrete CSF.
Where are the choroid plexuses located?	**The roofs of the third and fourth ventricles as well as on the floor and inferior horns of the lateral ventricles.**

Where is the main site of CSF absorption into the venous system?	**Arachnoid granulations are villi-like extensions of the arachnoid mater into the dural venous sinuses that are responsible for CSF absorption.**
Which dural reflection separates the right and left cerebral hemispheres? What are its attachments?	The falx cerebri can be found in the median-sagittal plane of the internal calvaria extending from the frontal crest and crista galli anteriorly to the internal occipital protuberance posteriorly.
Name the dural reflection located inferior to the tentorium cerebelli and its attachments.	The falx cerebelli is a vertical dural reflection that partially separates the cerebellar hemispheres. It extends from the tentorium cerebelli superiorly to the posterior cranial fossa inferiorly.
Which dural reflection separates the cerebral hemispheres from the cerebellum? What are its attachments?	The tentorium cerebelli attaches anteriorly to the clinoid processes of the sphenoid, laterally to the temporal bone, and posteriorly to the occipital/parietal bones.
What is the smallest dural in-folding and where is it located?	The diaphragma sella forms the roof over the hypophyseal fossa by anchoring on all four clinoid processes. It has a small aperture for the pituitary stalk (infundibulum) and hypophyseal veins.

Venous Sinuses and Flow (Figure 11.3)

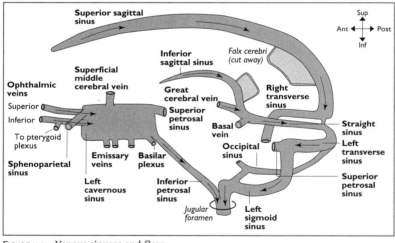

FIGURE 11.3 – Venous sinuses and flow.

Identify the following structures (Figure 11.4):

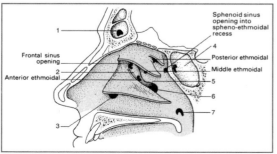

1. Frontal sinus
2. Hiatus semilunaris
3. Opening of nasolacrimal duct
4. Sphenoid sinus
5. Bulla ethmoidalis
6. Maxillary ostium
7. Eustachian ostium.

FIGURE 11.4 – Facial sinuses.

Identify the following structures (Figure 11.5):

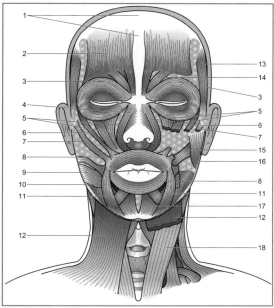

FIGURE II.5 – Facial musculature.

1. Epicranial aponeurosis
2. Frontal belly of occipitofrontalis m. (frontalis m.)
3. Orbicularis oculi m.
4. Nasalis m.
5. Levator labii superioris m.
6. Zygomaticus minor m.
7. Zygomaticus major m.
8. Orbicularis oris m.
9. Risorius m.
10. Depressor anguli oris m.
11. Depressor labii inferioris m.
12. Platysma m.
13. Temporalis m.
14. Corrugator supercilli m.
15. Buccinator m.
16. Masseter m.
17. Mentalis m.
18. Sternocleidomastoid m.

What are the muscles of mastication?   Masseter, temporalis, medial and lateral pterygoid mm.

Temporomandibular Joint (Figure 11.6)

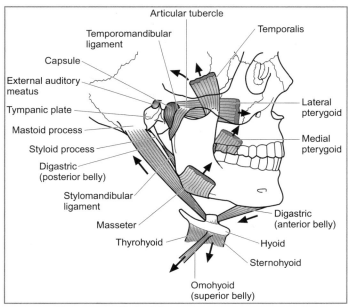

FIGURE II.6 – Temporomandibular joint.

CLINICAL ANATOMY

Name three sutures that are found in infants, but not in adults.	**Frontal suture, intermandibular suture, and intermaxillary suture.**
What is the remnant of the frontal suture known as in adults?	Metopic suture. It is important not to confuse it for a fracture on x-rays, because it does not fuse in 10% of the population.
What features predispose neonates to CN VII injury during prolonged deliveries that require instrumentation?	Absence of the mastoid process results in increased exposure of CN VII as it exits the stylomastoid foramen.
How many fontanelles can be found in a newborn?	Six (anterior, posterior, sphenoidal × 2, and mastoid × 2)
What clinical information can palpation of fontanelles deliver?	Bony growth of calvarium, hydration of infant, and intracranial pressure.
When are the anterior and posterior fontanelles no longer palpable?	**Anterior: 18 months old.** **Posterior: 12 months old.**
What is primary craniosynostosis?	Premature closure of skull sutures.
What is the most likely diagnosis in a patient with known head trauma who presents with a brief period of unconsciousness, followed by a lucid interval, and then unconsciousness once again?	**Epidural hematomas lead to relatively quick cerebral compression following a lucid interval. Most commonly, they are a result of head trauma involving damage to the middle meningeal a.**
What is the most likely diagnosis in a patient who complains of the "worst headache of my life" before losing consciousness?	**Subarachnoid hemorrhages typically result from rupture of arterial saccular aneurysms with extravasation of blood into the subarachnoid space.**
Is the hemorrhagic blood in subdural hematomas of arterial or venous origin?	**Subdural hematomas result from slower hemorrhage of blood from venous sinuses or bridging cerebral veins into the potential spaces of the dura.**
How can fractures to the pterion result in a fatal hematoma?	The pterion fracture may rupture the anterior branches of the middle meningeal artery that lie just deep to this landmark within the calvarium.
What nerve is commonly involved in patients with trigeminal neuralgia?	The sensory root of CN V (maxillary > mandibular > ophthalmic) with pain lasting 15 minutes or more in the respective sensory distribution.

Where are anesthetic agents injected during inferior alveolar nerve blocks in dental patients?	The mandibular foramen.
Weakness of unilateral facial muscles usually represents injury to what structure?	CN VII (facial nerve).
What are common causes of CN VII palsy?	Bell's palsy (idiopathic), exposure to cold, surgery, labor instrumentation, HIV infection, Lyme disease, and otitis media.

Match the following exam findings with the cranial nerve involved as shown in Figure 11.7:

Inability to open eyelids	CN III (C)
Hoarse voice after cardiac surgery	CN X (L)
Lack of gag reflex	CV IX (F)
Inability to smell oranges	CN I (H)
Unable to look down toward nose	CN IV (I)
Weakness when raising shoulders	CN XI (J)
Lack of vision in left eye	CN II (B)
Inability to clench teeth	CN V (K)
Not able to move eyes laterally	CN VI (D)
Vertigo/inability to hear commands	CV VIII (G)
Unilateral inability to raise eyebrows	CN VII (A)
Tongue deviates to left	CN XII (E)

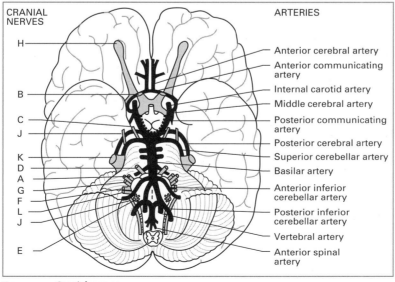

FIGURE 11.7 – Cranial nerves.

Infections of the facial veins within the "danger triangle of the face" may spread to the ___.

Cavernous sinus and pterygoid venous plexus (which are intracranial structures). Infection in these areas can injure surrounding nerves and vessels (Figure 11.8).

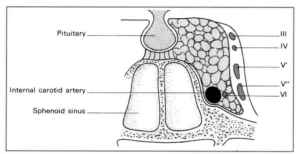

FIGURE 11.8 – Cavernous sinus.

List three general causes of hydrocephalus.

1. **Overproduction of CSF**
2. **Obstruction of CSF flow**
3. **Inability to absorb CSF**

What is the most common location for interference with CSF flow?

Cerebral aqueduct connecting the third and fourth ventricle.

Is the flow of CSF through the ventricles impaired in communicating hydrocephalus?

No, movement of CSF from the subarachnoid space to the venous system is blocked (↓ CSG absorption).

Failure of fusion of the lateral palatine processes, nasal septum, and/or the median palatine process results in what malformation?

Cleft palate.

Failure of fusion of what two processes results in cleft lip?

Maxillary and medial nasal processes.

Pain with pulling of the auricle is indicative of what infectious process?

Otitis externa.

What is the most likely diagnosis in a patient with a prominent red tympanic membrane with fluid in their middle ear?

Otitis media, usually from inflammatory blockage of the pharyngotympanic tube.

OSTEOPATHIC PRINCIPLES

What pre-ganglionic sympathetic nerves innervate the head and neck?

T1 to T4

What is the sensory innervation of the cranial dura mater?

CN V_1, CN V_2, CN V_3, C1, and C2.

What is the primary respiratory mechanism (PRM)?	An involuntary mechanical wave palpable in the cranium and throughout the body. The PRM is necessary for homeostasis and nervous system function. The PRM has two phases—inhalation and exhalation.
List the five phenomena of the PRM.	1. Motility (inherent motion) of the central nervous system (brain and spinal cord) 2. Fluctuation of CSF 3. Mobility (motion resulting from surrounding structures) of intracranial and intraspinal membranes 4. Articular mobility of cranial bones 5. Involuntary mobility of the sacrum between the ilia. *Note: To better understand Motility vs. Mobility, see Chapter13: Abdominal and Pelvic Viscera—Osteopathic Principles and Practices.*
Describe the two phases of the PRM.	**1. Inhalation phase: Flexion of midline bones and external rotation of paired bones leading to increased transverse diameter and decreased A–P and vertical diameters.** **2. Exhalation phase: Extension of midline bones and internal rotation of paired bones leading to decreased transverse diameter and increased A–P and vertical diameters.**
What is the cranial rhythmic impulse (CRI)?	Besides circulation, the CSF exhibits an inherent rhythmic fluctuation known as the CRI. It is a cyclical movement of the CSF often described as a tide or wave.
What is the "Breath of Life"?	Dr. Wm. G. Sutherland called the potency or energy within the CSF that drives the CRI the "Breath of Life." The breath of life is qualitative, while CRI is quantitative.
What is the normal rate of the CRI?	**10–14 cycles per minute. The CRI decreases in frequency and amplitude in states of disease.**
What is the reciprocal tension membrane (RTM)?	The RTM is formed by the falx cerebri, tentorium cerebelli, and falx cerebelli. With attachments to anterior, superior, lateral, posterior, and inferior poles of the cranium, the RTM is under constant tension in all three planes. Any change of shape in one plane is accommodated with a complementary change in the other planes.

What is the Sutherland fulcrum?	The tension in the RTM converges along the straight sinus where all four dural folds meet forming a physiologic fulcrum. This fulcrum is suspended, automatically shifting as the shape of its attachments change, maintaining balance in the RTM.
Describe the involuntary craniosacral motion exhibited by the sacrum between the ilia.	**Unlike postural flexion and extension (middle transverse axis), craniosacral motion of the sacrum occurs along an axis through S2. Craniosacral flexion causes the base of the sacrum to move posterior (counternutation). Craniosacral extension causes the base of the sacrum to move anterior (nutation).**

 Memory Aid: Postural (middle transverse axis) and Cranial (superior transverse axis) flexion/extension are opposite to each other.

Note: The superior transverse axis for respiratory motion of the sacrum also passes through S_2. Many sources consider the craniosacral and superior transverse axes to be one axis allowing both respiratory and craniosacral flexion/extension.

Describe the connection between the cranium and the sacrum.	The inner layer of the dura mater continues in to the spinal canal. This layer of dura has firm attachments to the foramen magnum, dens and posterior portions of the vertebral bodies of C_2, C_3, and S_2.
What is the sphenobasilar symphysis (SBS)?	**The articulation between the basisphenoid and the basiocciput, a reference point for cranial motion and a key articulation in physiologic and non-physiologic dysfunction (A.K.A. sphenobasilar synchondrosis or junction).**

DIAGNOSIS

What are clues indicating possible craniosacral dysfunction?	**Any history of trauma to the head or sacrum is a strong indication to look for cranial dysfunctions. Patients presenting with migraines, neuropsychiatric complaints, low back (lumbosacral region) pain, stress, genetic diseases, or after dental procedures may also have cranial dysfunctions.**

In neonates, prolonged/difficult parturition, decreased feeding/suckling, vomiting, drowsiness, irritability, colicky behavior, etc. are signs of craniosacral dysfunction.

Describe the following holds:	*In the following holds, the patient is supine and the examiner is seated comfortably at the patient's head. It is important to maintain very light pressure.*
Vault hold	Using both hands, the physician's fingers are spread to contact the patient's head as follows:
	Second digit on greater wing of sphenoid;
	Third digit anterior to ear (squamous portion of temporal bone);
	Fourth digit behind the ear (mastoid process);
	Fifth digit reaches toward occiput across occipitomastoid suture; and
	Thumbs should not contact patient so that no pressure is transmitted to cranium via thumbs.
Fronto-occipital hold	One hand cups the patient's occiput from below and the other hand rests across the forehead with thumb and fourth (or fifth) digit over the greater wings of the sphenoid.
Temporal bone (Becker) hold	Using loosely interlaced fingers, cup the patient's occiput with thumbs reaching behind the ears over the mastoid processes.
What is the difference between physiologic and non-physiologic dysfunctions?	Physiologic dysfunctions are a result of restrictions that exist while still allowing SBS flexion/extension and craniosacral inhalation/exhalation. They are often asymptomatic.
	Non-physiologic dysfunctions restrict SBS flexion/extension and craniosacral inhalation/exhalation. They are most commonly a result of direct or indirect trauma to the head or sacrum.

Physiologic Craniosacral Dysfunctions (Table 11.2)

TABLE II.2 – Physiologic Craniosacral Dysfunctions

Dysfunction at SBS	Effect on SBS	Effect on Sphenoid	Effect on Occiput
Flexion	The SBS shows better freedom with motion into flexion than extension.	Axis: Transverse through the body Flexion > Extension	Axis: Transverse above the foramen magnum Flexion > Extension
Extension	The SBS shows better freedom with motion into extension than flexion.	Axis: Transverse through the body Extension > Flexion	Axis: Transverse above the foramen magnum Extension > Flexion
Left torsion	Along the AP axis, the SBS will appear **twisted**.	Axis: AP through the center of the body The **left** greater wing of the sphenoid will rotate **upward**.	Axis: AP through the center of the sphenoid body The **left** half of the occiput will rotate **down** (opposite direction to sphenoid).
Right torsion (Figure 11.9)	Along the AP axis, the SBS will appear **twisted**.	Axis: AP through the center of the body The **right** greater wing of the sphenoid will rotate **upward**.	Axis: AP through the center of the sphenoid body The **right** half of the occiput will rotate **down** (opposite direction to sphenoid).

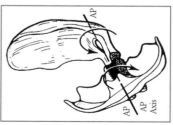

FIGURE II.9 – Right torsion.

156

Dysfunction at SBS	Effect on SBS	Effect on Sphenoid	Effect on Occiput
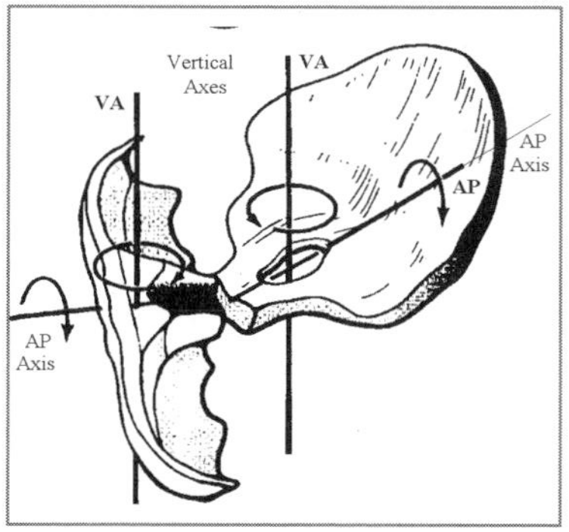 Left sidebending and rotation (Figure 11.10)	The SBS will sidebend to the left along vertical axes (shifting the SBS slightly to the left and creating a left-sided convexity) as well as rotate left along an AP axis.	Axes: 1. Vertical through center of body; 2. AP through center of body. Along the vertical axis, the base shifts left; the left greater wing moves anterior. Along the AP axis, the left greater wing moves inferior.	Axes: 1. Vertical through center of foramen magnum; 2. AP through center of sphenoid body. Along the vertical axis, the basilar (anterior) part shifts left; the left half moves posterior (opposite the sphenoid). Along the AP axis, the left half moves inferior (same as the sphenoid).

FIGURE 11.10 – Left sidebending and rotation.

Right sidebending and rotation	The SBS will sidebend to the right along vertical axes (shifting the SBS slightly to the right and creating a right-sided convexity) as well as rotate right along an AP axis.	Axes: 1. Vertical through center of body; 2. AP through center of body. Along the vertical axis, the base shifts right; the right greater wing moves anterior. Along the AP axis, the right greater wing moves inferior.	Axes: 1. Vertical through center of foramen magnum; 2. AP through center of sphenoid body. Along the vertical axis, the basilar (anterior) part shifts right; the right half moves posterior (opposite the sphenoid). Along the AP axis, the right half moves inferior (same as the sphenoid).

AP, Anteroposterior; SBS, sphenobasilar symphysis or synchondrosis.

157

TABLE 11.3 – **Non-Physiologic Craniosacral Dysfunctions**

Dysfunction at SBS	Effect on SBS	Mechanism of Injury
Superior vertical strain	The SBS is not properly aligned in the sagittal plane. The sphenoid (body) is displaced **superior** in relation to the occiput (Figure 11.11). FIGURE 11.11 – Superior vertical strain.	Traumatic blow to the bottom of the face/jaw.
Inferior vertical strain	The SBS is not properly aligned in the sagittal plane. The sphenoid (body) is displaced **inferior** in relation to the occiput.	Traumatic blow to the top of the face/frontal bones or fall on the sacrum.
Left lateral strain	The SBS is not properly aligned in the transverse plane. The sphenoid (body) is displaced to the **left** in relation to the occiput.	Any injury to the right side of the forehead or face.
Right lateral strain	The SBS is not properly aligned in the transverse plane. The sphenoid (body) is displaced to the **right** in relation to the occiput (Figure 11.12). FIGURE 11.12 – Right lateral strain.	Any injury to the left side of the forehead or face.
Compression	The SBS is compressed. The sphenoid is pushed posteriorly into the occiput (Figure 11.13). FIGURE 11.13 – Compression.	Any midline injury from the front of the face or back of the head in an AP direction.

Note: Non-physiologic dysfunctions may be superimposed over physiologic dysfunctions.
AP, Anteroposterior; SBS, sphenobasilar symphysis or synchondrosis.

What is the difference between interosseous lesions and intraosseous lesions?

Interosseous lesions are dysfunctions found across a joint or articulation of two or more bones.

Intraosseous lesions are dysfunctions found within a single bone, between two different regions or ossification centers.

How is the temporo-mandibular joint (TMJ) evaluated?

Thorough evaluation of the TMJ includes:

1. **Clicks or restrictions with opening and closing of the jaw**
2. **Active and passive elevation, depression, protrusion, retraction, and lateral deviation**
3. **Internal and external rotation with the PRM of temporal and mandibular bones (paired bones).**

TREATMENT

Differentiate between occipito-atlantal joint (OA) compression and condylar compression.

OA compression involves locking and restriction between the occiput and atlas (C_1). It is an interosseous lesion.

Condylar compression is a dysfunction within the occipital condyles—intraosseous lesion. Each occipital condyle is formed from two separate ossification centers—basilar process and condylar part. A force across these two parts of the occipital condyles can lead to condylar compression.

What is a still point?

It is a fulcrum created by balancing osseous and membranous tissue tension. The "Breath of Life" is used best through a still point to correct a dysfunction.

Describe the following craniosacral treatment methods.

CV_4 (Compression of the fourth ventricle)

The supra occiput is gently compressed to decrease the amplitude of inhalation (SBS flexion) and exaggerate exhalation (SBS extension). This pressure compresses the posterior cranial fossa and fourth ventricle while pushing the cerebellum anterior toward the foramen magnum and brainstem. Once a still point is achieved, the PRM is negligible. The PRM is no longer resisted and allowed to return. Full return of the PRM completes the treatment. The parietals, temporals, or sacrum may also be used for a CV_4.

Results: ↑ frequency, amplitude, and symmetry of the CRI throughout the body. Regain autonomic nervous system and fluid homeostasis. Induce uterine contractions for labor.

Remember: When all else fails, use a CV_4.

Lift and V-spread techniques	Both techniques are used to disengage sutures and balance membranous tension. Lifts are most commonly performed on the frontal and parietal bones using a gentle and diffuse grip to distract superiorly. For a V-spread, the index and middle fingers are placed on either side of a suture (e.g., occipitomastoid suture) to spread and disengage the underlying suture.
OA decompression	Using the SP of C_2 and the posterior basiocciput as levers, gently pull them away from each other in a superior-inferior direction. This distracts the occipital condyles away from the atlas.
	Due to the proximity of the jugular foramen to the OA, this can be used to treat problems pertaining to the internal jugular v. and CNs IX, X, and XI.
Condylar decompression	Place the tips of the last three digits of both hands in the suboccipital region superior to C_2. Apply a pressure directed superiorly toward the basiocciput and anteriorly, to disengage the condyles from the atlas. Balance the intraosseous tension in the occipital condyles and basiocciput until an intraosseous release is felt and the PRM is stronger.
	The jugular foramen lies lateral to the occipital condyles at the junction of the basilar process and condylar part of the occiput. Indications thus, are similar to that of OA decompression.
Venous sinus drainage	Must perform a thoracic inlet release and OA or condylar decompression before cranial venous drainage. Venous sinuses must be drained in an inferior to superior fashion beginning with the occipital and transverse sinuses and ending with the superior sagittal sinus. Sinus drainage is achieved by spreading overlaying sutures apart using techniques such as the V-spread or using crossed thumbs over a suture to distract the sutures laterally and away from each other.
What techniques may be used in treatment of TMJ syndrome?	After finding restrictions in motion of the TMJ, gentle passive stretch and muscle energy techniques may be the most effective. Counterstrain to ligaments such as the temporo-mandibular or stylo-mandibular ligaments may provide relief. Craniosacral treatment of the mandible and temporal bones may also be used.
What is the Galbreath technique?	A passive soft tissue technique to improve drainage of the inner ear via the eustachian tube and lymphatics.

How is the Galbreath technique performed?	With the patient seated or supine, the physician stabilizes the patient's forehead using one hand. The fingers of the other hand are placed over the superior ramus of the mandible with the fingertips at the TMJ. The mandible is gently adducted and the TMJ is distracted/disengaged using mild antero-inferior (approximately 55 degrees below horizon) traction.
What are the primary applications of the Galbreath technique?	It is effective for the treatment of infections of the ears, nose, or throat.
What is the significance of the use of the Galbreath technique in the pediatric patient population?	Due to the smaller head size of pediatric patients, the eustachian tube has a more horizontal position. This results in decreased drainage of the middle ear leaving the child at a higher risk for developing otitis media. The Galbreath technique improves drainage via the eustachian tube by increasing the vertical orientation of the eustachian tube. Spreading the sutures bilaterally at the zygomas, frontals, and mandibles away from the temporals also gives significant relief.

SECTION V

Thoracic, Abdominal, and Pelvic Viscera

CHAPTER 12 THORACIC VISCERA

GROSS ANATOMY OVERVIEW

Identify the labeled structures on the chest film (Figure 12.1):

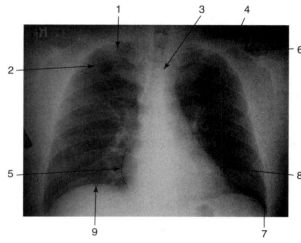

1. Posterior rib
2. Anterior rib
3. Carina
4. Clavicle (left)
5. Right heart border
6. Scapula
7. Costo-phrenic angle
8. Left heart border
9. Right hemidiaphragm over liver

FIGURE 12.1 – Chest radiograph (PA view).

Chest Radiograph (lateral view) (Figure 12.2)

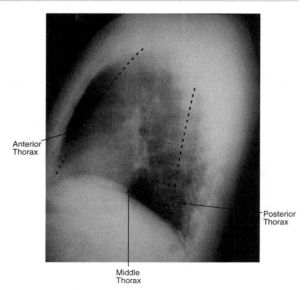

Anterior Thorax

Posterior Thorax

Middle Thorax

FIGURE 12.2 – Chest radiograph (lateral view).

Surface Anatomy of the Lungs (Figure 12.3)

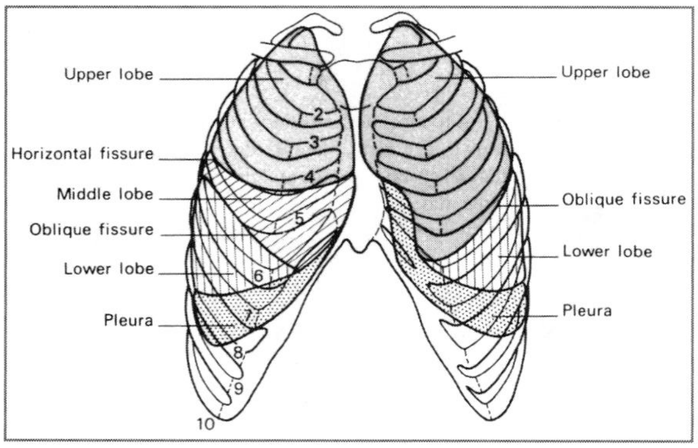

FIGURE 12.3 – Surface anatomy of the lungs.

What is the difference between visceral and parietal pleura?	Visceral pleura intimately invests the outer surface of the lungs (including lobes and fissures) whereas the parietal pleura is an interior lining of the thoracic wall.
What is the pleural cavity and what does it contain?	It is the potential space between the visceral and parietal pleura and it contains serous pleural fluid.
What is the location of the right pulmonary artery in relation to the right main bronchus? How about on the left side?	**R**ight pulmonary artery is **A**nterior to right main bronchus. The **L**eft pulmonary artery is **S**uperior to left main bronchus. *Memory Aid:* **RALS**: **R**ight → **A**nterior, **L**eft → **S**uperior
What is the homolog of the right middle lobe in the left lung?	The lingula.
Name the arteries that solely supply nutrition to the tissues of the lung.	The bronchial arteries.
Where do the bronchial arteries arise?	Left bronchial artery ← thoracic aorta. Right bronchial artery ← superior posterior intercostal artery, third posterior intercostal artery, and/or left superior bronchial artery.
What structures carry the oxygenated blood from the lungs to the left atrium?	**The pulmonary veins.**
How is the pericardium bound to the abdominal diaphragm?	**The pericardiophrenic ligament attaches the pericardium to the central tendon of the diaphragm.**

What are the two layers of the pericardium?	External → Fibrous pericardium Internal → Serous pericardium (parietal and visceral)
What are the first two branches of the aorta?	Right and left coronary arteries.
What are the best locations to identify the cardiac veins? Where do they all drain?	Great cardiac v. → anterior interventricular groove Middle cardiac v. → posterior interventricular groove Small cardiac v. → accompanying marginal a. They all drain into the coronary sinus.

Identify the labeled heart structures (Figure 12.4):

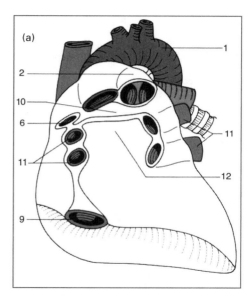

1. Aorta
2. Pulmonary trunk
3. Right ventricle
4. Cusps of aortic valve
5. Left ventricle
6. Superior vena cava
7. Fossa ovale
8. Coronary sinus
9. Inferior vena cava
10. Transverse sinus
11. Pulmonary veins
12. Oblique sinus

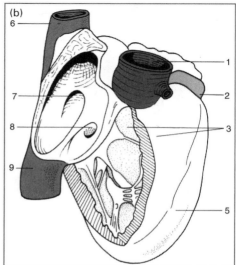

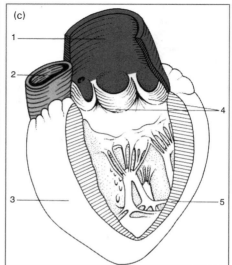

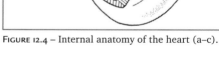

FIGURE 12.4 – Internal anatomy of the heart (a–c).

What structures drain into the right atrium?	Superior vena cava, inferior vena cava (IVC), and coronary sinus.
What structures do the recurrent laryngeal nerves loop around as they ascend to the larynx?	**Right: right subclavian artery** **Left: arch of aorta/ligamentum arteriosum**

Coronary Circulation (Figure 12.5)

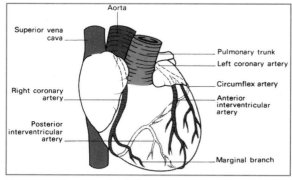

FIGURE 12.5 – Coronary circulation.

Thoracic Arteries (Figure 12.6)

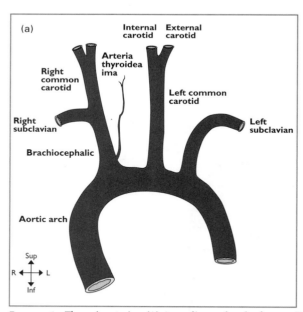
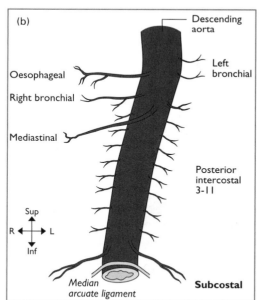

FIGURE 12.6 – Thoracic arteries. (A) Ascending and arch of aorta; (B) thoracic (descending) aorta; (C) arterial anastomoses around scapula.

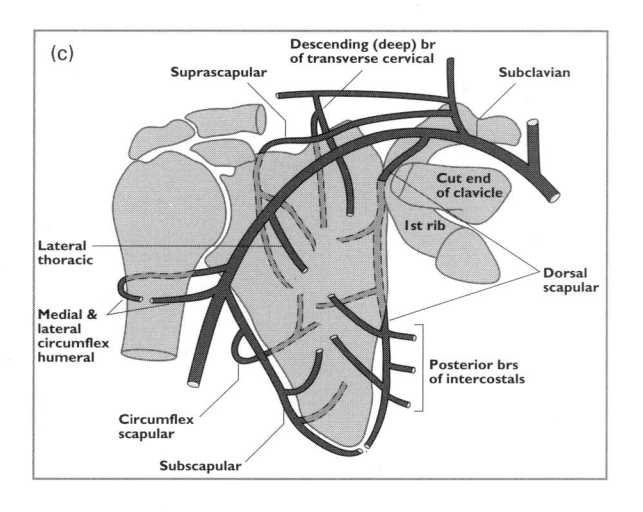

FIGURE 12.6 – *Continued*

List the major arteries that supply the breast.

Internal thoracic, lateral thoracic, thoracoacromial, and posterior intercostal aa.

Thoracic Venous Drainage (Figure 12.7)

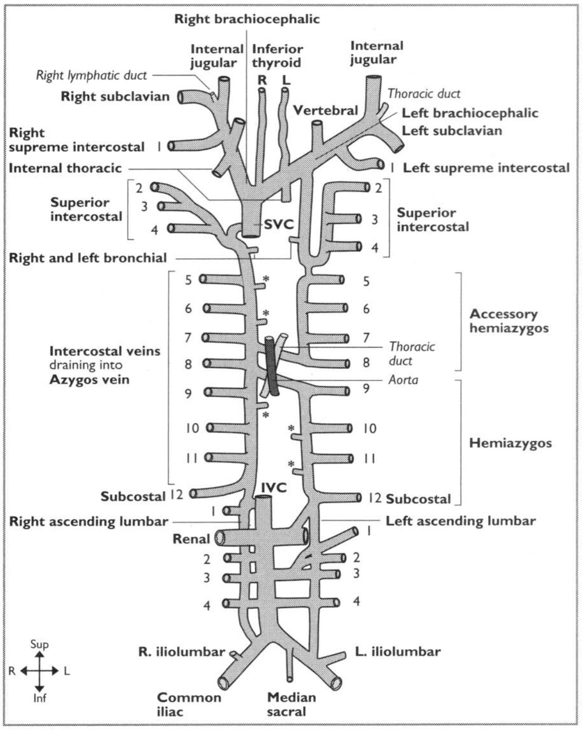

FIGURE 12.7 – Thoracic venous drainage.

Thoracic Lymph Glands (Figure 12.8)

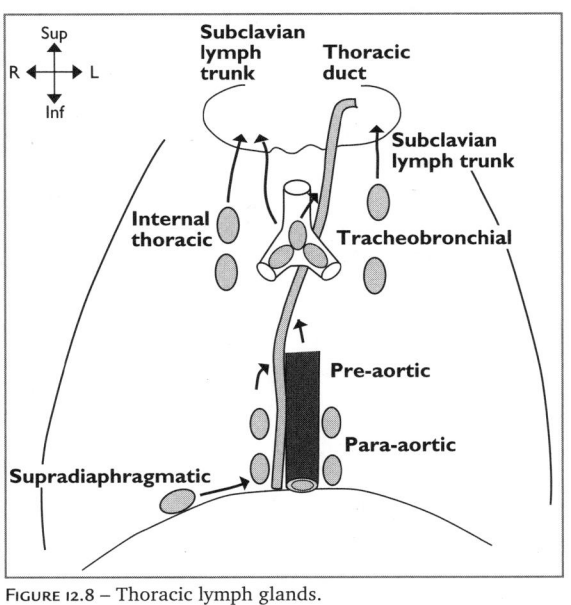

FIGURE 12.8 – Thoracic lymph glands.

Thoracic Lymphatic Drainage (Figure 12.9)

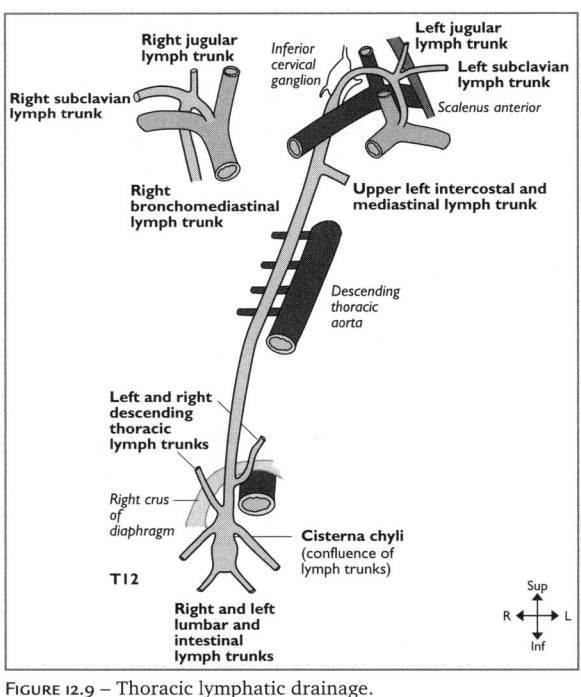

FIGURE 12.9 – Thoracic lymphatic drainage.

What structures pass through the diaphragm at the levels of T_8, T_{10}, and T_{12}?

IVC/Right Phrenic n.: T_8
T_{10}: Esophagus/Vagus nn.
Aorta/Azygos v./Thoracic duct: T_{12}.

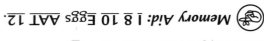 **Memory Aid: I 8 10 Eggs AAT 12.**

CLINICAL ANATOMY

What is the path of lymphatic drainage for the breast?

Subareolar lymphatic plexus → anterior axillary, posterior axillary, infraclavicular, and internal thoracic groups.

In what quadrant of the breast is carcinoma most common?

The upper-outer quadrant.

What is on the top of one's differential diagnoses in a patient complaining of shortness of breath status-post central venous catheterization?

Pneumothorax (air collecting in the pleural cavity) is a well-known complication of this procedure.

What is the difference between a pneumothorax, a hydrothorax, and a hemothorax?

Pneumothorax: air in pleural cavity.
Hydrothorax: fluid collecting in pleural cavity.
Hemothorax: blood collecting in pleural cavity.

What is a likely diagnosis when a pleural rub is heard on auscultation of the lungs?

Pleuritis (pleurisy) resulting from inflammation of the pleura.

What are the four most common anterior mediastinal masses?

Thyroid goiter, Thymoma, Teratoma, Terrible lymphoma.
Memory Aid: 4 T's.

After swallowing a shirt button, a child presents with difficulty breathing. On auscultation, on what side do you expect to hear decreased breath sounds?

The right side because the right mainstem bronchus has a steeper vertical angle that is more conducive to lodging foreign bodies.

A child presents after swallowing a quarter. How, using plain x-ray study, would you confirm the location of the quarter?

With use of an AP x-ray of the neck and chest.
- If the quarter is lodged in the esophagus, the quarter will appear flat as the muscular esophagus collapses flat into the coronal plane.
- If the quarter is lodged in the trachea, a cross-section of the quarter will be visible as the cartilaginous trachea has a greater diameter anterior to posterior than from left to right.

After remaining stationary for an 18-hour flight, a passenger complains of shortness of breath. What is a likely etiology that must be evaluated immediately?

Pulmonary thromboembolism, most likely from a deep venous thrombosis. A ventilation/perfusion scan or pulmonary arterial angiogram can be ordered.

What cardiac sinus do surgeons identify in order to set up a cardiopulmonary bypass?

Transverse pericardial sinus because it allows access to the aorta and pulmonary trunk.

What is an ideal location to perform a pericardiocentesis (draining the pericardial cavity)?

Place a wide-bore needle into the inferior aspect of the left parasternal fifth or sixth intercostal space.

In emergent cases, a subxiphoid approach with a wide-bore needle at the left xiphocostal angle, $\frac{1}{2}$ cm below the costal margin pointing toward the left shoulder is used.

Fetal Circulation (Figure 12.10)

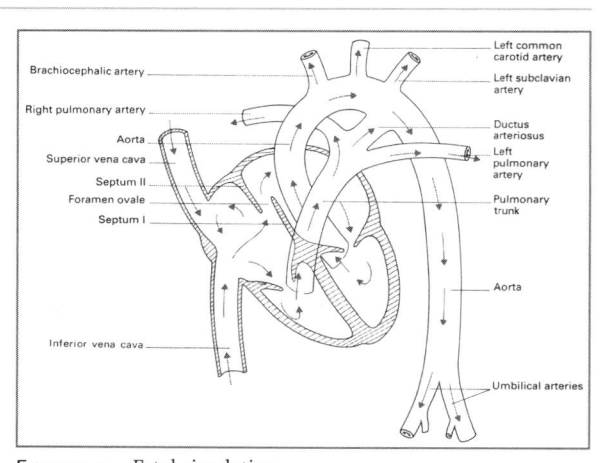

FIGURE 12.10 – Fetal circulation.

Congenital Malformations of the Heart (Figure 12.11)

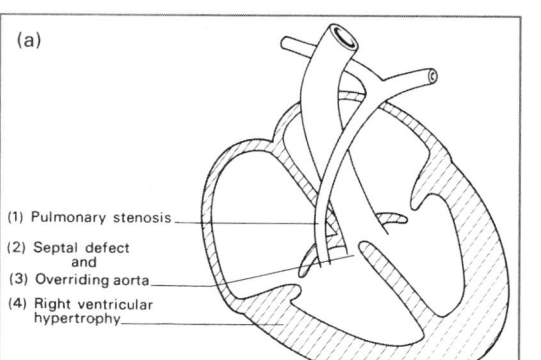
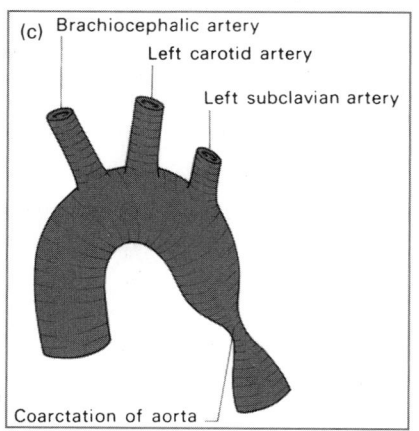

FIGURE 12.11 – Congenital malformations of the heart. (a) Tetralogy of Fallot; (b) patent ductus arteriosus; (c) coarctation of the aorta.

After cardiac surgery, a patient complains of hoarseness. What structure is likely to have been injured during the surgery?

The left recurrent laryngeal n. as it loops around the arch of the aorta and ligamentum arteriosum.

Injury to what nerves passing lateral to the pericardium can be fatal?

The phrenic nerves (C3, C4, C5) on their way to innervate the diaphragm.

 Memory Aid: C3, 4, 5 keeps the diaphragm alive.

What is a tracheo-esophageal fistula?

Congenital malformation most commonly seen as a blind upper esophageal pouch with a fistula between the lower esophagus and the trachea at around T_4 (Figure 12.12).

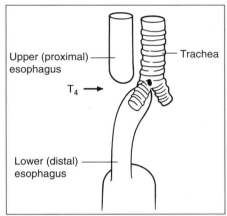

FIGURE 12.12 – Tracheoesophageal fistula.

OSTEOPATHIC PRINCIPLES AND PRACTICES

What pre-ganglionic sympathetic nerves innervate the following organs? List the effects of sympathetic stimulation.

Trachea and bronchi	**T1–T5** **Bronchodilation; thickened mucous production; increased number of goblet cells.**
Esophagus (distal ⅔)	**T1 or T2–T6 or T8** **Decreased peristalsis; increased tone of lower esophageal sphincter**
Lungs	**Vasoconstriction; decreased lymphatic flow.**
Lung parenchyma	**T1–T6**
Lung visceral pleura	**T1–T7**
Lung parietal pleura	**T1–T11**

Heart	T1–T5 or T6 (T2 on the left is the most commonly affected)
Coronary vasculature	Decreased blood flow secondary to vasoconstriction.
SA node, AV node	Increased rate (leading to tachyrhythmias)
Myocardium	Increased oxygen demand secondary to ↑ inotropy and ↑ chronotropy.

What nerve delivers parasympathetic innervation to the thoracic viscera?	Vagus nerve (CN X).

What are the effects of increased parasympathetic innervation on:

Trachea and bronchi	Bronchoconstriction; increased (thin-watery) mucous production.
Esophagus (distal $\frac{2}{3}$)	Increased peristalsis; lower esophageal sphincter relaxation.
Lungs	Vasodilation; decreased lymphatic spasm.
Coronary vasculature	Increased blood flow secondary to vasodilation.
Sinoatrial node, A-V node	Decreased rate (possibly leading to bradyrhythmias or heart blocks).
Myocardium	Decreased oxygen demand.

What are the four categories for restrictions of the thorax and associated viscera?	1. Osteoarticular (vertebrae, ribs, sternum, etc.) 2. Muscular (intercostal, neck, diaphragm, etc.) 3. Fascial (mediastinal, pleura, pericardial, suspensory, etc.) 4. Visceral.

Describe the suspension of the lungs in the thoracic cavity.	The parietal pleura lines the thoracic cavity and has several myofascial and ligamentous attachments to the thoracic cage. Of osteopathic importance are the pleural attachments to the lower cervical and upper thoracic vertebrae, rib 1, manubrium, sternum, and diaphragm. These attachments form the major suspensory/support system of the lungs and affect their function significantly.

How is the heart suspended in the thoracic cavity?	Bands of loose connective tissue form the superior and inferior sternopericardial ligaments connecting the pericardium to the sternum at the sternal angle and xiphoid process, respectively. The superior sternopericardial ligament is the primary suspension of the heart. The pericardial sac is also continuous with the central tendon of the diaphragm (via the cardiophrenic ligament) and esophageal connective tissue.

How are restrictions of the visceral tissues and organs discovered?

"Listening" techniques. An examiner places their hands gently over the region being examined. The examiner projects their palpation to the internal tissue being examined and "listens" for stress patterns, areas of strain or restriction and regions of increased/decreased heat.

How are visceral organs treated using osteopathic manipulation?

Once an area requiring treatment is discovered, a physician may use indirect or direct treatments.

Indirect Tx: take the tissue into the freedom.

Direct Tx: take the tissue into its barrier/restriction away from the freedoms.

Treatment may also be directed to the regions of autonomic innervation and ligamentous attachments to the musculoskeletal system.

Describe treatment of the sternum.

Sternal release: With the patient lying supine, physician places one hand over the sternum and one hand below the thorax with digits pointing caudally. For every motion induced by the anterior hand, the posterior hand induces the opposite motion. Sternal motion is tested for vertical, lateral, and torsional strains. After finding the freedoms, treatment may be delivered to the sternum via direct or indirect technique.

What is a sternal lift?

In addition to being a point of convergence for the thoracic cage, the sternum has a strong effect on the mediastinum, pericardium, and pleura due to connective tissue attachments. Using one finger from each hand as hooks on the manubrium and xiphoid process, the physician lifts the sternum anteriorly and waits for release or change in tissue tension.

CHAPTER 13

ABDOMINAL AND PELVIC VISCERA

GROSS ANATOMY OVERVIEW

Abdominal Surface Anatomy (Figure 13.1)

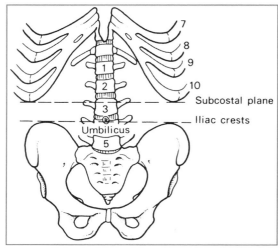

FIGURE 13.1 – Abdominal and pelvic surface anatomy.

What bony structures can be used to describe the margins of the following organs?

Liver	**Ribs 5 to 10 on the right**
Spleen	**Ribs 9 to 11 on the left**
Gallbladder	Tip of ninth costal cartilage on the right
Neck of pancreas	Transpyloric plane (level of L1)
Kidneys	**Right: L1 to L3**
	Left: T12 to L2

Identify the labeled structures of abdominal wall (Figure 13.2):

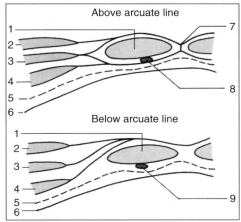

FIGURE 13.2 – Rectus sheath.

1. Rectus abdominis m.
2. External oblique m.
3. Internal oblique m.
4. Transversus abdominis m.
5. Transversalis fascia
6. Peritoneum
7. Linea alba
8. Superior epigastric a.
9. Inferior epigastric a.

Identify the labeled structures (Figure 13.3):

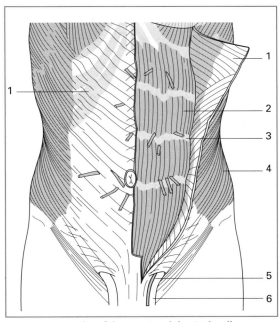

FIGURE 13.3 – Muscles of the anterior abdominal wall.

1. Anterior rectus sheath
2. Rectus abdominis m.
3. Tendinous intersection
4. External oblique m.
5. Ilioinguinal n.
6. Spermatic cord

Lumbar Plexus (Figure 13.4)

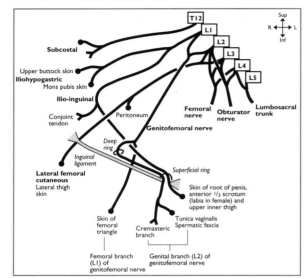

FIGURE 13.4 – Lumbar plexus.

Sacral Plexus (Figure 13.5)

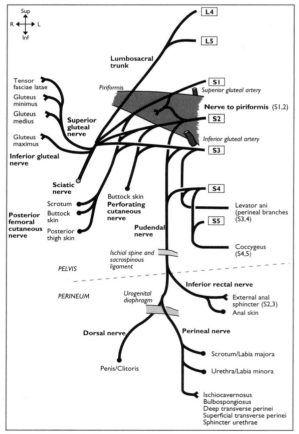

FIGURE 13.5 – Sacral plexus.

What layer of peritoneum invests intimately with the stomach?	Visceral peritoneum invests the outer surfaces of viscera such as the stomach whereas parietal peritoneum lines the internal surface of the abdominal and pelvic walls.
The lesser omentum connects the liver to what structures?	The lesser curvature of the stomach and proximal duodenum.
An axial (transverse cross) section through the greater omentum would reveal how many layers of peritoneum?	Four: A double layer of peritoneum hanging like an apron from the greater curvature of the stomach and then folding back up to the transverse colon.

Mesentery (Figure 13.6)

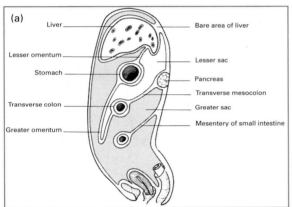
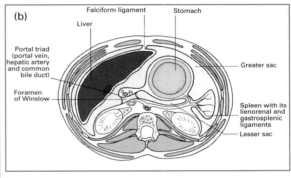

FIGURE 13.6 – Mesentery. (a) Longitudinal section of peritoneal cavity; (b) transverse section of peritoneal cavity.

What is the most posterior extent of the peritoneal cavity?	Morrison's pouch (hepatorenal recess).
Describe the three embryonic divisions of the gastrointestinal tract?	**Foregut: Mouth → Ampulla of Vater.** **Midgut: Ampulla → distal $\frac{1}{3}$ of transverse colon.** **Hindgut: Distal $\frac{1}{3}$ of transverse colon to anus.**
What organs are considered retroperitoneal?	**K**idneys and ureters, **I**nferior Vena Cava, **D**escending Colon, **A**scending Colon, **A**drenal Glands, **A**orta, **R**ectum, **P**ancreas, **S**econd, third, and fourth parts of the Duodenum. ***Memory Aid:*** **KID**neys **A**nd **A**drenals **A**re **R**etro-**P**eritoneal **S**tructures.

Arteries of the Abdomen and Pelvis (Figure 13.7)

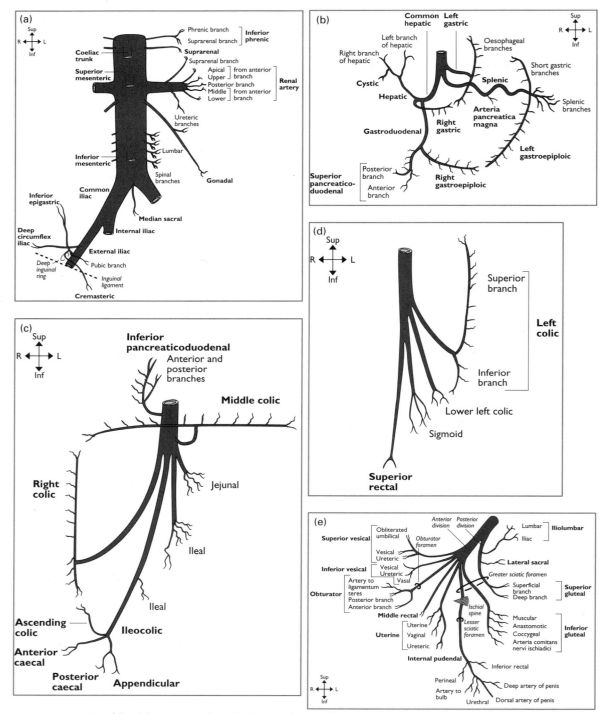

FIGURE 13.7 – Arteries of the abdomen and pelvis. (a) Abdominal aorta; (b) celiac trunk; (c) superior mesenteric artery; (d) inferior mesenteric artery; (e) internal iliac artery.

Venous Drainage of the Abdomen and Pelvis
(Figure 13.8)

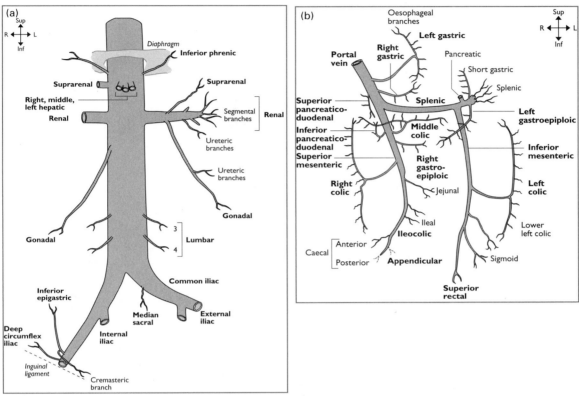

FIGURE 13.8 – Venous drainage of the abdomen and pelvis. (a) Inferior vena cava; (b) portal vein.

Lymph Nodes of the Abdomen and Pelvis (Figure 13.9)

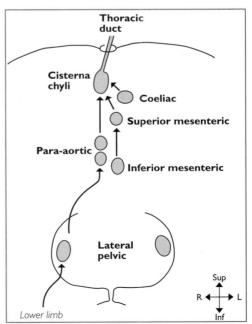

FIGURE 13.9 – Lymph nodes of the abdomen and pelvis.

Autonomics of the Abdomen and Pelvis (Figure 13.10)

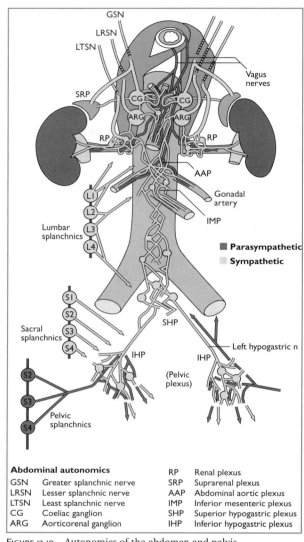

Abdominal autonomics			
GSN	Greater splanchnic nerve	RP	Renal plexus
LRSN	Lesser splanchnic nerve	SRP	Suprarenal plexus
LTSN	Least splanchnic nerve	AAP	Abdominal aortic plexus
CG	Coeliac ganglion	IMP	Inferior mesenteric plexus
ARG	Aorticorenal ganglion	SHP	Superior hypogastric plexus
		IHP	Inferior hypogastric plexus

FIGURE 13.10 – Autonomics of the abdomen and pelvis.

Which vagus nerve travels anteriorly in the abdomen?   The left vagus n.

Spermatic Cord and Layers (Figure 13.11 and Table 13.1)

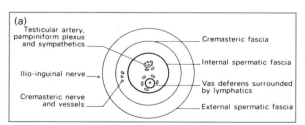

FIGURE 13.11 – Spermatic cord and testes. (a) Contents of spermatic cord; (b) inguinal rings; (c) transverse section of testes.

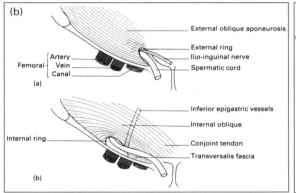

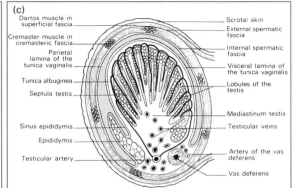

Figure 13.11 – *Continued*

Table 13.1 – Spermatic Cord and Layers

Abdominal Wall	Spermatic Cord	Scrotum/Testes
Skin	Skin	Scrotum and septum
Subcutaneous tissue	Dartos (superficial) fascia and muscle	Scrotum and septum
External oblique aponeurosis	External spermatic fascia	External spermatic fascia
Internal oblique muscle and fascia	Cremaster muscle and fascia	Cremaster muscle and fascia
Transverse abdominal muscle	Does not continue into spermatic cord	Does not continue into scrotum
Transversalis fascia	Internal spermatic fascia	Internal spermatic fascia
Peritoneum	Tunica vaginalis	Obliterated processus vaginalis

What are the borders of the following triangles:

Calot's triangle   Cystic duct, common hepatic duct, cystic a.

Hesselbach's triangle   **Inguinal ligament, epigastric vessels, lateral border of rectus sheath**

How is the liver connected to the following structures:

Anterior abdominal wall   Falciform ligament

Stomach   Gastrohepatic ligament*

Duodenum   Hepatoduodenal ligament*

Combined, these two ligaments comprise the lesser omentum.

Identify the labeled structures in the liver (Figure 13.12):

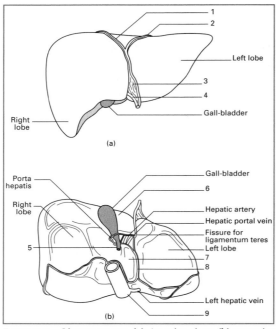

(a)

(b)

FIGURE 13.12 – Liver anatomy. (a) Anterior view; (b) posterior view.

1. Coronary ligament
2. Triangular ligament
3. Falciform ligament
4. Round ligament of liver (ligamentum teres hepatic)
5. Common bile duct
6. Quadrate lobe of liver
7. Quadrate lobe of liver
8. Fissure for ligamentum venosum
9. Inferior vena cava (IVC)

What is Cantle's line?

A line drawn from the IVC to the left of the gallbladder fossa separating the right and left lobes of the liver.

Relations of the Spleen (Figure 13.13)

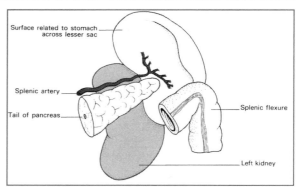

FIGURE 13.13 – Relations of the spleen.

Identify the labeled regions of the stomach (Figure 13.14):

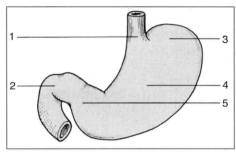

FIGURE 13.14 – Stomach anatomy.

1. Cardia
2. Pyloric sphincter
3. Fundus
4. Body of stomach
5. Pyloric antrum

Identify the labeled structures (Figure 13.15):

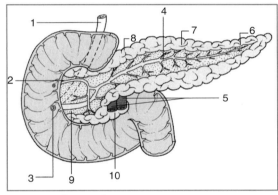

FIGURE 13.15 – Pancreatic anatomy.

1. Common bile duct
2. Accessory pancreatic duct (of Santorini)
3. Duodenal papilla
4. Main pancreatic duct (of Wirsung)
5. Superior mesenteric vessels
6. Tail of pancreas
7. Body of pancreas
8. Neck of pancreas
9. Head of pancreas
10. Uncinate process of pancreas

What are three characteristics that can be used to distinguish the jejunum from the ileum?	1. Jejunum has longer vasa recta 2. Jejunum has a few larger arcade loops 3. Jejunum has closely packed plicae circulares
List the differences between the small bowel and colon?	Teniae coli, haustra, and appendices epiploicae can all be found on the colon.
What is an easy visual technique that can be used to locate the appendix?	Follow the teniae coli until they converge at the base of the cecum.
What is the most common location of the appendix?	Retrocecal.

How can one distinguish the transverse colon from the ascending and descending colon during colonoscopy?

The lumen of the **Tr**ansverse colon appears **Tri**angular due to the three ligamentous attachments to the transverse colon:

1. Transverse mesocolon posteriorly
2. Gastrocolic ligament superiorly
3. Greater omentum anteriorly.

 Memory Aid: **Tr**ansverse colon has a **Tri**angular lumen.

Relations of the Kidney (Figure 13.16)

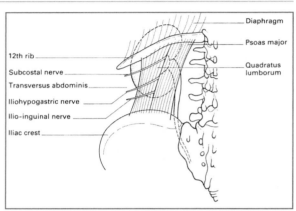

FIGURE 13.16 – Relations of the kidney.

What structures cross directly over the ureters?

Uterine artery (in ♀) *or* ductus deferens (in ♂).

Where does the left ovarian vein drain?

Left renal v. (Right ovarian v. drains into IVC.) The same holds true for testicular vv. in males.

What fascia surrounds the kidney?

Gerota's fascia.

Identify the labeled structures (Figure 13.17):

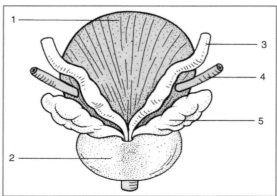

FIGURE 13.17 – Posterior view of the bladder.

1. Bladder
2. Prostate
3. Vas deferens
4. Ureter
5. Seminal vesicle.

What is the innervation to the prostate?

Parasympathetics—pelvic splanchnic nerves (S2–S4).

Sympathetics—inferior hypogastric plexus (L1, L2).

Identify the labeled structures of the pelvis
(Figure 13.18):

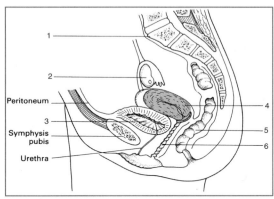

FIGURE 13.18 – Longitudinal section of female pelvis.

1. Sacral promontory
2. Ovary and fallopian tube
3. Bladder
4. Uterus
5. Rectum
6. Vagina

Identify the labeled structures of the uterus
(Figure 13.19):

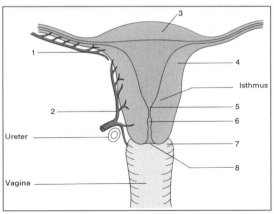

FIGURE 13.19 – Coronal section of uterus.

1. Ovarian a.
2. Uterine a.
3. Fundus of uterus
4. Body of uterus
5. Internal os
6. Cervical canal
7. Lateral fornix
8. External os.

What structures are contained in the following
ligaments of the uterus:

Broad ligament	Round ligament, fallopian tube.
Round ligament	No important structures.
Suspensory ligament of ovaries	Ovarian vessels.
Transverse cervical ligament	Uterine vessels.

What is the name for the space between the
bladder/uterus and rectum?

Pouch of Douglas.

187

What is the embryonic significance of the pectinate (dentate) line?	This line marks the division between the ectoderm and endoderm derived anus.
What arteries supply the penile erectile tissue?	Dorsal and deep dorsal artery. The dorsal artery arises from the internal pudendal artery and travels on the dorsum of the penis deep to buck's fascia. The two deep dorsal arteries travel within the corpora cavernosa.

CLINICAL ANATOMY

List the layers of the anterior abdominal wall that a surgeon would traverse from superficial to deep.	1. Camper's fascia (superficial and fatty) 2. Scarpa's fascia (deeper and membranous) 3. Anterior rectus sheath 4. Rectus abdominis m. 5. Posterior rectus sheath 6. Transversalis fascia 7. Peritoneum.
What is the general term for developmental abnormalities that lead to abdominal structures entering the thorax?	Diaphragmatic hernia. Most common: Sliding (type I) hiatal hernia (95%): Cardia/gastroesophageal junction slides up, regurgitation symptoms. Paraesophageal (type II) hiatal hernia: Fundus is caught in the hiatus, no regurgitation symptoms. Type III: Combined type I and II. Type IV: Other abdominal organs herniate through diaphragmatic defect.
In a patient with alcoholic cirrhosis, collateral circulation via the portosystemic anastomoses will manifest with what symptoms?	**1. Bleeding esophageal varices** **2. Hemorrhoids** **3. Caput medusae (around umbilicus)**
Cessation of breathing or pain when pressure is placed in the right subcostal margin indicates what pathology?	Acute cholecystitis (this is known as Murphy's sign).
What structure is most likely to be injured in a stab wound to the left tenth intercostal space?	Spleen.
Which artery is the most common source of bleeding in duodenal ulcers?	**Gastroduodenal artery.**
Describe McBurney's point.	$\frac{1}{3}$ the distance from the anterior superior iliac spine to the umbilicus, estimates the position of the appendix.

Are hemorrhoids above the pectinate line more painful than those below?	No, internal hemorrhoids (above the line) have visceral innervation and are not painful. External hemorrhoids (below the line) have somatic innervation (painful).
Describe the characteristics of an indirect inguinal hernia.	A hernia passing through the deep and superficial inguinal rings, lateral to Hesselbach's triangle, and presenting as a bulge in the scrotum.
A patient presenting with an anterior abdominal wall bulge medial to the inferior epigastric vessels most likely has what abnormality?	Direct inguinal hernia through Hesselbach's triangle.
Where can one palpate the superficial inguinal ring?	Superolateral to the pubic tubercle.
What are the major complications of cryptorchidism (undescended testes)?	Infertility and potential for malignancy.
If an enlarged scrotal sac transilluminates with a light pen, what is the most likely diagnosis?	Hydrocele of the testis.
A patient who presents with a dilated and tortuous pampiniform plexus on ultrasound is most likely suffering from a ____.	Varicocele.
What structure is bilaterally excised in a vasectomy?	Ductus deferens.
Which gender is more prone to developing urinary tract infections (UTIs)?	Males in their infancy, and females during most of their lives.
Why are male infants more prone to developing UTIs than female infants?	Male infants are prone to lower urinary tract obstruction due to a congenital anomaly known as posterior urethral valves. This obstruction can lead to stasis and reflux of urine, predisposing them to UTIs.
Why are females more prone to developing UTIs later on in life?	The short urethras, internalization of the urethra, and the absence of prostatic fluid (which has some antimicrobial quality), all increase the chance of bacterial colonization.

Name the following kidney congenital abnormalities (Figure 13.20):

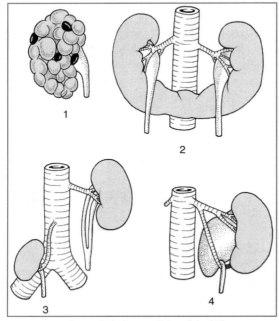

FIGURE 13.20 – Congenital abnormalities of the kidney.

1. Polycystic kidney
2. Horseshoe kidney
3. Ectopic pelvic kidney (with duplicate ureter)
4. Aberrant renal a. (with hydronephrosis).

Other renal abnormalities include bifid/duplicate renal pelvis, retrocaval ureter, uni- or bilateral renal agenesis and supernumerary kidney.

When will Lloyd's punch test be positive?

Kidney infection and/or posterior peritoneal irritation.

Note: Lloyd's punch test is positive when gentle tapping of a seated patient's costovertebral angle elicits pain.

What is the lymphatic drainage of the prostate gland?

Lymphatic drainage from the prostate is to the internal iliac and sacral lymph nodes.

Where are the five locations along the ureter that are prone to obstruction from a calculus?

1. Ureteropelvic junction
2. External iliac vessels at the pelvic brim
3. Juxtaposition between vas deferens and ureters
4. As the ureter angulates anteromedially
5. Ureterovesicular junction.

Where does urine extravasate in the following injuries?

Fracture of bony pelvis

Rupture of intermediate part of urethra → deep perineal pouch

Rupture of bulb of penis

Rupture of spongy urethra → superficial perineal space

OSTEOPATHIC PRINCIPLES AND PRACTICES

What pre-ganglionic sympathetic nerves innervate the following organs? List the effects of sympathetic stimulation.

Stomach and duodenum (proximal)	T5–T9 (left) via greater splanchnic n. to celiac ganglion. Decreases gastric emptying and peristalsis, constricts pylorus, reduces secretions.
Intestinal tract	T5–L2 Decreases peristalsis, constriction of all sphincters.
Midgut: duodenum (distal), jejunum, ileum, appendix, ascending colon and transverse colon (proximal ⅔)	T10–T11 or T12 via lesser splanchnic n. to superior mesenteric ganglion.
Hindgut: transverse colon (distal ⅓), descending colon, sigmoid colon, and rectum	T12–L2 via least splanchnic n. (T12) and lumbar splanchnic n. (L1–L2) to inferior mesenteric ganglion.
Appendix	T10 or T12 (right)
Liver	T5–T9 (many argue the liver has no sympathetic innervation). Glycogenolysis.
Gallbladder and ducts	T5–T7 (right) Lumenal relaxation with sphincter contraction.
Pancreas	T7 Decreases secretory function.
Spleen	T7 (left) Vasoconstriction.
Adrenal glands	T10–T11 Medullary secretion of catecholamines.
Kidneys	T10–T11 Vasoconstriction, decreased glomerular filtration rate (GFR), ↑ renin secretion.
Ureters	Proximal ureters: T10–T11 or T12 Distal ureters: T12–L1 or L1–L2 Decreased peristalsis.
Urinary bladder and urethra	T12–L2 Detrusor m. relaxation, sphincter constriction.
Prostate gland or uterus/cervix	T10 or T12–L2 Constriction/contraction of uterus, relaxation of cervix. Unknown effect on prostate gland.
Testes or ovaries	T10–T11 Vasoconstriction.
Penis or clitoris	T12–L2 Ejaculation.

What nerve delivers parasympathetic innervation to the following organs? What are the effects of increased parasympathetic innervation on:	
Stomach and duodenum (proximal)	Vagus n. Increases gastric emptying and peristalsis, pyloric relaxation, increases secretions.
Intestinal tract	Vagus n. and sacral plexus (pelvic splanchnic) nn. (S2–S4) Increases peristalsis, relaxation of all sphincters.
Midgut: duodenum (distal), jejunum, ileum, appendix, ascending colon and transverse colon (proximal ⅔)	Vagus n.
Hindgut: transverse colon (distal ⅓), descending colon, sigmoid colon, and rectum	S2–S4
Liver	Vagus n. Glycogenesis and gluconeogenesis.
Gallbladder and ducts	Vagus n. (right) Lumenal contraction with sphincter relaxation leading to lumenal emptying.
Pancreas	Vagus n. Increases secretory function.
Spleen	Vagus n. (left) Vasoconstriction.
Adrenal glands	None
Kidneys	Vagus n. Vasodilation, increased GFR.
Ureters	Proximal: Vagus n. Distal: S2–S4 Increased peristalsis.
Urinary bladder and urethra	S2–S4 Detrusor m. contraction, sphincter relaxation.
Prostate gland or uterus/cervix	S2–S4 Relaxation of uterus, constriction of cervix. No or unknown effect on prostate gland.
Testes or ovaries	Vagus n. Unknown effects.
Penis or clitoris	S2–S4 Erection.
Where can somatic dysfunction be found in patients with acute appendicitis?	T_{10} or T_{12}. On many occasions, the Chapman's point for the appendix on the lateral tip of the right rib 12 is tender.

What motions do visceral organs exhibit?	1. Visceral mobility 2. Visceral motility.
What is the difference between visceral mobility and motility?	Visceral mobility is the motion exhibited by viscera as result of surrounding organs, structures, muscles, ligaments, and bones. Visceral motility is the inherent and characteristic motion created by the organ itself. Motility tends to be a repetitive pendulum-like motion moving back and forth between "inhalation" and "exhalation" positions (different than those of respiration and craniosacral motions).
What factors contribute to visceral mobility?	1. Motion via the somatic (voluntary) nervous system (resulting from voluntary motions of the musculoskeletal system) 2. Motion via the autonomic (involuntary) nervous system (resulting from involuntary motions such as respiration and cardiac contractions) 3. Motion via craniosacral inhalation and exhalation.
Is peristalsis of the gastrointestinal (GI) tract considered visceral mobility or motility?	Peristalsis is considered motility of the GI tract itself, as it is generated and acting on the GI tract itself. However, the motion induced in adjacent organs by peristalsis would be mobility of these adjacent organs.
How are osteopathic dysfunctions of the viscera described?	Restrictions, resistance, or barriers in the motion of the mobility or motility of the viscera are used to describe osteopathic dysfunctions of the visceral organs.
How are osteopathic dysfunctions of the viscera discovered?	Passively, superficial and/or deep palpation (based upon location of organ) and "listening" techniques can help judge the motion of the viscera. Active motion testing by moving the organs in all planes of its motion may also be used to discover restrictions.
How can sympathetic innervation via the celiac, superior mesenteric and/or inferior mesenteric ganglia be normalized?	These ganglia are located midline, evenly spaced between the xiphoid process and umbilicus. With the patient supine, posteriorly directed pressure along the line connecting the xiphoid process and umbilicus can be used to inhibit the tissue until a release or tissue texture changes are felt. Thus, sympathetic flow through these ganglia may be normalized.

What modalities may be used to treat restrictions in visceral mobility and motility?

1. Direct techniques
2. Indirect techniques
3. Induction.

Describe treatment using direct techniques.

When treating the viscera, maintaining a gentle touch is very important. When a restriction is found, the physician moves the organ in a manner to engage the barrier and gradually allow it to gently pass through the barrier. Any excessive or inappropriate force may cause damage to the viscera and its surrounding tissues.

How are indirect techniques performed in visceral manipulation?

Once again, a gentle touch is the most therapeutic. The organ is moved in its direction of ease or freedom, away from the adhesion or barrier. This will gradually allow the organ to "disengage" from its barrier or resistance and return to its normal mobility and motility.

What is induction?

Induction techniques primarily treat visceral dysfunctions dealing with motility. To appropriately deliver treatments using induction, a thorough knowledge of the organ's inherent motion (motility) and its axis is necessary. The physician gently assists both the "inhalation" and "exhalation" phases of the organ's motility to restart and revitalize the organ's internal "drive."

SECTION VI

Osteopathic Approach to Specialties

14 FAMILY MEDICINE

MIGRAINE HEADACHE

What is the most common type of migraine headache?	**Migraine without aura.**
What are the criteria for diagnosis of migraine without aura?	Headache lasting 4 to 72 hours, throbbing headache, moderate to severe in intensity, usually unilateral, worse with exertion, nausea, vomiting, photophobia, phonophobia.
What are the most common triggers of migraine headaches?	Stress, hormonal fluctuations, vasodilatory medications, alcohol, cheese, wine, foods containing tyramine and monosodium glutamate.
What is the common age of first migraine?	**Between 15 and 25 years old.**
What are the indications for neuroimaging in migraine?	Focal neurologic deficits, atypical headache pattern, headache worse with Valsalva maneuver, rapid worsening symptoms, new onset in older patient, awakening from sleep.
What is the role of the trigeminovascular system in migraine?	Activation of this system by an insult to the brain occurs, which releases vasoactive peptides producing pain and vasodilation.
What structures are supplied by CN V that may be involved in headache?	1. Dura 2. Cerebral arteries
What effect of the sympathetics activates the trigeminovascular system?	Vasoconstriction leads to decreased blood flow to the brain. This activates the trigeminovascular system, leading to vasodilation and pain.
What nerves converge on the trigeminal tract?	Spinal nerves C1–C3; CN V, VII, IX, and X. Afferent pain stimuli from these nerves can trigger the trigeminovascular system.

SINUSITIS

What are the most common causes of sinus drainage obstruction?	**Viral upper respiratory infection and allergic rhinitis.**
What are common non-infectious causes of sinusitis?	Rhinitis, polyps, foreign bodies, swimming, immune deficiency, anatomic anomalies.
What are the most common signs and symptoms of sinusitis?	Erythematous and congested nasal mucosa, halitosis, anosmia, postnasal drip, headache, purulent nasal discharge, fever, dull throbbing pain, and tenderness over involved sinus.
What sinuses are most commonly infected?	Ethmoid and maxillary.
What is the most common presenting head pain associated with sinusitis for each location?	1. Maxillary: Toothache, frontal headache 2. Frontal: Frontal headache 3. Ethmoid: Pain behind and between the eyes, splitting frontal headache 4. Sphenoid: Not well localized, referred pain to frontal and occipital areas.
What should be suspected in a nursing home patient with a nasogastric tube?	**Occult sinusitis.**
What are the complications of infection spreading from the ethmoidal sinuses?	Blindness and optic neuritis via spread through wall adjacent to orbit.
What adjacent structures can be affected by extension of sphenoid sinusitis?	Optic nerve and carotid artery.
What is the main anatomic reason for the increased likelihood of maxillary sinusitis?	The ostia is located high on the superior medial walls of the maxilla.
What sensation is common with inflammation of the maxillary sinus mucous membranes?	Sensation of toothache of the molars. Both areas are innervated by CN V_2.
What are the effects of hypersympathetic tone on the respiratory epithelium?	**Increased number of goblets cells leading to production of thick sticky secretions.**
What are the effects of sphenopalatine ganglion stimulation on the sinuses?	Parasympathetic effects: Profuse, clear, thin secretions.
Somatic dysfunctions of what areas are commonly associated with sinusitis?	**Occipito-atlantal joint (OA), cervical spine (C_1–C_2) and soft tissue hypertonia, clavicles, cervicothoracic junction.**

What are the goals of OMT in sinusitis?	1. Relieve obstruction and pain
	2. Improve lymphatic and venous drainage
	3. Improve mucociliary clearance
	4. Alter somatovisceral reflexes to sinuses.

OTITIS MEDIA

What is the most common age of occurrence for otitis media?	Between 3 months and 3 years old.
What are the common signs and symptoms of otitis media?	Ear pain, fever, conductive hearing loss, bulging, dull appearing, erythematous tympanic membrane with indistinct landmarks, bubbles or air fluid levels, displaced light reflex.
What factors predispose to acute otitis media?	Nasopharyngeal infection, eustachian tube dysfunction.
What is a sign of persistent effusion?	Painless hearing loss.
What is the most common sequela to acute otitis media?	Serous otitis media.
What should be suspected if tenderness to palpation over mastoid process is present in a patient with otitis media?	**Mastoiditis. The mucosal lining of the middle ear is continuous with that of the mastoid cells.**
What does drainage or purulent material emanating from the middle ear indicate?	Perforation of the tympanic membrane or concomitant otitis externa.
What anatomic differences of the eustachian tube increase the susceptibility to middle ear infections in children?	**Eustachian tube is shorter and more horizontal and narrower than in adults.**
What role does inflammation of the adenoids play in otitis media?	It can occlude the eustachian tube, facilitating migration and growth of pathogens.
What are the effects of increased sympathetic tone?	**Increased vasoconstriction, which leads to decreased lymphaticovenous drainage and nutrient supply to tissues.**
What is the lymphatic drainage of the middle ear?	**Deep parotid or upper deep cervical lymph nodes.**
What exercises can clear middle ear effusion?	Swallowing and chewing.

199

List nerves that may refer pain to the middle ear and cause otalgia.	**CN V, VII, IX, and X, and upper cervical nerves**
What disorders commonly refer pain to the middle ear?	1. Dental abscess 2. Temporomandibular disorder

PHARYNGITIS

What are the common causes of pharyngitis?	Viral and bacterial infections, allergies, irritants.
What are the complications of group A Streptococcus *pharyngitis?*	Acute rheumatic fever, glomerulonephritis, peritonsillar and retropharyngeal abscesses.
What is the classic presentation on physical exam of the throat for group A strep?	**Palatal petechiae with strawberry tongue (also fever, lymphadenopathy, rash, and exudates).**
Describe the rash associated with group A strep throat.	Diffuse red-bluish rash, sandpaper texture, blanches with pressure, desquamates in 1 week especially over the palms and soles. Starts on the trunk and spreads peripherally.
What is the lymphatic drainage for the pharynx?	Lymph drains to the jugulodigastric node, from there to the inferior deep cervical nodes.
Where is jugulodigastric node located?	Posterior to the ramus of the mandible.
What are the effects of increased sympathetic tone on the pharynx?	Vasoconstriction decreasing the ability to mount immune response, inhibits secretions, decreases lymphatic and venous drainage.
What are common areas of somatic dysfunctions associated with pharyngitis?	**Suboccipital, clavicles, hyoid, cervical and upper four thoracic vertebrae.**

ASTHMA

What are the characteristics of asthma?	Reversible episodic airway obstruction, airway inflammation, hypersensitivity of the bronchial tree to a variety of stimuli.
What are the main features of bronchial asthma?	Abnormally strong spasmodic contractions of the bronchial smooth muscles, edema of airway mucosa, increased mucus secretions, cellular infiltration, and desquamation of airway epithelium.
What is the primary determinant factor of airflow resistance?	Radius of the conducting airways.

What are the primary muscles of inspiration?	**Diaphragm, external intercostals, and interchondral part of internal intercostals.**
What are some of the accessory muscles of inspiration?	**Scalenes, sternocleidomastoid.**
What factors increase the work of breathing?	Decreased pulmonary compliance, increased airway resistance, decreased elastic recoil of lungs, and limited mechanical motion of the rib cage, diaphragm, and adjacent structures.
What is the effect of somatic dysfunction of the thoracic cage?	**Decreased compliance of the thoracic cage.**
What are the parasympathetic effects on the airways?	Production of profuse thin secretions, vasodilation, bronchiole constriction, increased airway resistance.
What are the sympathetic effects on the airways?	Thickening of secretions, bronchiole dilatation, increased airway radius, decreased airway resistance and vasoconstriction.
What are common somatic dysfunctions found with asthma?	**T_1–T_6 paraspinal muscles (especially T_3–T_4 on the left), C_2, ribs, diaphragm, sternum, clavicles.**
Which osteopathic manipulative techniques should be avoided during an acute asthma attack?	Direct stimulation of OA, C_1–C_2, which may activate vagal induced bronchospasm.
What areas should be the focus of OMT in asthma patients?	Mobilization of thoracic cage, clavicle, diaphragm, sternum and paraspinal tissues, in both acute and chronic stages of asthma.
What is the predominant rib cage dysfunction in asthma?	**Inhalation dysfunction**

HYPERTENSION

What effect does prolonged hypertension have upon the baroreflexes?	It resets the baroreflexes (aortocarotid and cardiopulmonary) to a higher blood pressure.
What is the action of baroreflexes on sympathetic outflow?	Inhibition of sympathetic nervous system outflow.
What are the hypersympathetic effects on the heart?	Supraventricular arrhythmias, ventricular fibrillation, increased force of contraction, vasoconstriction, coronary vasospasm, and cardio-acceleration.

What are the effects of decreased sympathetic tone on the heart?	Decreased venous capacity and decreased ability to develop collateral circulation.
What are the hyperparasympathetic effects on the function of the heart?	Cardio-deceleration, A-V blocks, hypotension, decreased force of contraction, predisposition to bradycardia.
What are the Chapman's reflex points for the heart?	**1. Anterior: second intercostal space, between second and third ribs near the sternum.** **2. Posterior: intertransverse space between T_2–T_3, midway between the spinous and transverse processes.**
What is the lymphatic drainage for the heart?	**Tracheobronchial lymph nodes usually on the right side.**
What is the effect of impaired lymphatic drainage?	Increased central venous pressure, increased tissue congestion, decreased nutrient delivery.
What is the effect of hypersympathetic tone on kidney function?	Vasoconstriction of the afferent arteriole to the kidney, decreased glomerular filtration rate and urine output, increased release of antidiuretic hormone and aldosterone, retention of fluids and electrolytes.

CONSTIPATION/DIARRHEA

What is the definition of constipation?	**Delayed transit of intestinal contents, resulting in less than three stools per week, however individual differences exist.**
What are the causes of constipation?	Low-fiber diets, dehydration, sedentary lifestyle, emotional stress, medications (opioids, antacids, iron, diuretics, antihistamines, antidepressants).
Constipation is a presenting symptom in what disease processes?	Irritable bowel syndrome, ulcerative proctitis, rectal fissures or abscesses, rectal strictures, obstructive disorders.
What medications are used to treat constipation?	Laxatives, stool softeners.
How can OMT be used to enhance bowel movements?	Treating the autonomic nervous system ($\uparrow$ parasympathetics and $\downarrow$ sympathetics) will help stimulate peristalsis. Sacral rocking and opening up the sacroiliac (SI) joint are also helpful. *Remember: always start with opening up the pelvic diaphragm.*

What are the requirements for passage of stool and defecation?	1. Increased intra-abdominal pressure
	2. Relaxation of sphincters and pelvic floor
	3. Opening of rectal canal
	4. Adequate stool volume, colonic motility, and a patent colon
What is diarrhea?	**Increase in stool weight greater than 250 g in 24 hours.**
What are the mechanisms leading to diarrhea?	Osmotic load within intestine, excessive secretion of electrolytes and water into intestinal lumen, exudation of protein and fluid from intestinal mucosa, and altered intestinal motility.
What are the effects of increased sympathetic tone on the colon?	Decreased peristalsis, constipation, symptoms of ileus, increased sphincter tone, abdominal distention, flatulence.
What are the effects of increased parasympathetic tone upon the colon?	Increased peristalsis, diarrhea, increased glandular and enzyme secretion, relaxation of sphincter tone.
What is the dominant autonomic nervous system in a patient with diarrhea?	**The parasympathetic nervous system is responsible for increased motility of the intestinal system.**
What OMT techniques can be used to treat the symptoms of diarrhea?	Treatment of the OA (OA decompression) and sacrum (sacral rocking, SI joint release) work to normalize parasympathetic tone. Normalizing sympathetic (rib-raising) will also help.
What is the location of specific Chapman's reflex points anteriorly along the iliotibial band?	1. **Cecum: Right greater trochanter**
	2. **Sigmoid colon: Left greater trochanter**
	3. **Hepatic flexure: Right lateral epicondyle**
	4. **Splenic flexure: Left lateral epicondyle.**

LOW BACK PAIN

What muscles are commonly involved in low back pain (LBP)?	Erector spinae, gluteus maximus, abdominals, hamstrings, iliopsoas.
What is spondylolisthesis?	Forward slippage of one vertebra over another.
What is spondylolysis?	Defect or stress fracture of the pars interarticularis (posterior arch of vertebra).
What is spondylosis?	Degenerative changes in the intervertebral disc and annulus.

What is spinal stenosis?	Narrowing of the spinal canal.
What is the neurologic testing for spinal nerve L4?	**Dorsiflexion of the foot, knee jerk, and sensation testing to medial calf.**
What is the neurologic testing for spinal nerve L5?	**Dorsiflexion of the great toe and sensory to medial forefoot. No specific spinal reflex.**
What is the neurologic testing for spinal nerve S1?	**Eversion of the foot, ankle jerk, and sensation to lateral foot.**
What is straight leg raise test?	Test for disc herniation and sciatic nerve irritation.
What is suspected with LBP accompanied by inability to heel-to-toe walk or squat/rise?	**Cauda equina injury (incontinence may also be seen).**
What is suspected with point tenderness on palpation or percussion of the spine?	Fracture, infection, neoplasm of the spine.
What is suspected with pain elicited upon extension of the spine?	Consider spinal stenosis.
What is suspected with pain elicited upon flexion of the spine?	Mechanical causes of LBP.
What is psoas syndrome?	**Bilateral psoas spasm with one side more prominent than the other leading to LBP.**
What is iliolumbar ligament syndrome?	**Referred pain from a tense iliolumbar ligament to the sacroiliac joint, inguinal ligaments, pubes or femoral triangle.**
What is posterior facet syndrome?	Referred pain from a tear in the capsule of the posterior zygapophyseal joints to the buttocks and posterior thigh.

CHAPTER 15 INTERNAL MEDICINE

PULMONARY MEDICINE: PNEUMONIA

What are the signs and symptoms of pneumonia?	Cough with sputum, fever, and shortness of breath.
What is the osteopathic manipulative approach to the treatment of pneumonia?	Rib-raising to increase rib motion and normalize sympathetics. Lymphatic techniques to decrease congestion. Correcting thoracic and sternal restrictions also decreases the work required to breathe. Release of the occipito-atlantal joint (OA) and atlanto-axial joint (AA) as well as correcting cervical somatic dysfunctions will normalize parasympathetics by treating the vagus nerve.
What is the most common rib dysfunction in patients with pneumonia?	**Exhalation dysfunction (thought to be due to repetitive coughing).**
Which aspect of the osteopathic treatment of a patient with pneumonia should be addressed first?	Treat hypersympathetic tone first.
What role does hypersympathetic tone play in pneumonia?	**Increases the thickness of mucus, decreases arterial and venous supply to the lungs, and decreases lymphatic flow from the lungs.**
What osteopathic treatment is relatively contraindicated?	High velocity low amplitude (HVLA)

PULMONARY MEDICINE: CHRONIC OBSTRUCTIVE PULMONARY DISEASE

Describe asthma.	Reversible obstructive lung disease characterized by airway inflammation, increased bronchial secretions, and bronchial smooth muscle constriction caused by hyper-responsiveness. It can affect people of all ages, but is commonly seen in children. It may or may not have an allergic component, but there is usually a precipitating event such as an infection or hypersensitivity.
What are common signs and symptoms of asthma?	Episodes of dyspnea, expiratory wheezing, and cough are common. Use of accessory muscles of respiration indicates increased severity.

205

What somatic dysfunction(s) is typically found in asthma?	**Third or fourth rib somatic dysfunction.**
What are the diagnostic criteria for chronic bronchitis?	A patient must have a productive cough for at least 3 months over 2 consecutive years.
Describe emphysema.	Emphysema is an irreversible lung disorder, which is characterized by destruction of alveoli and airway dilatation distal to the terminal bronchiole.
Describe bronchiectasis.	It is an irreversible pathologic dilation of the bronchioles in response to a toxin.
What are common signs and symptoms of bronchiectasis?	Hemoptysis, cough with sputum, and wheezing. Bacterial colonization often occurs because of the secretions and tissue injury.
What are the two osteopathic components of chronic obstructive pulmonary disease?	1. Mechanical component: impaired rib motion that may be due to rib somatic dysfunction, diaphragm restriction, or fascial restrictions.
	2. Physiologic component: hypersympathetic tone can increase the thickness of secretions and cause vasoconstriction of the lung tissue. Hyperparasympathetic tone can lead to excessive watery secretions. Impaired lymphatics can lead to congestion.

PULMONARY MEDICINE: CYSTIC FIBROSIS

Describe cystic fibrosis.	It is an autosomal recessive disease (chromosome 7) that produces an abnormal protein called cystic fibrosis transmembrane regulator. It leads to an abnormal chloride channel, which causes secretion of thick mucus that creates obstruction in the lungs and other organs. This dysfunction allows for increased infections and colonization of the lungs. Patients with cystic fibrosis also have increased incidence of sinusitis and nasal polyps. Diagnosis is aided by the chloride sweat test.
What osteopathic techniques would aid in the treatment of cystic fibrosis?	**Thoracic pump and releasing the diaphragm to mobilize mucus, rib-raising to increase rib motion and normalize sympathetics (decrease thickness of mucus), and sinus drainage for sinusitis.**

CARDIOVASCULAR: ANATOMY AND OSTEOPATHIC PRINCIPLES

What are the parasympathetics to the heart?	Vagus n. (CN X)
What portion of the heart does the right vagus n. innervate?	The right vagus nerve innervates at the sinoatrial (SA) node. **Memory Aid:** **SARA** (**SA** node: **R**ight-sided **A**utonomics).
What portion of the heart does the left vagus n. innervate?	The left vagus nerve innervates the atrioventricular (AV) node. **Memory Aid:** **LAVA** (**L**eft-side: **AV** node **A**utonomics).
How do the parasympathetics work on the heart?	**The parasympathetics are negatively chronotropic and therefore slow the rate of contraction.**
What do the parasympathetics do to the vasculature?	**Vasodilate the vasculature.**
What are the effects of increased parasympathetic tone?	1. Bradyarrhythmias via innervation of the SA node 2. Heart block via innervation of the AV node 3. Hypotension and diminished vital organ perfusion
What spinal nerves are responsible for the sympathetic innervation of the heart?	**T1–T5 or T6.**
What parts of the heart do the right-sided sympathetics predominantly innervate?	The right heart and SA node. **Memory Aid:** **SARA** (**SA** node: **R**ight-sided **A**utonomics).
What parts of the heart do the left-sided sympathetics predominantly innervate?	The left heart and the AV node. **Memory Aid:** **LAVA** (**L**eft-side: **AV** node **A**utonomics).
How does the sympathetic nervous system affect the heart?	**The sympathetics are positive inotropes and chronotropes; therefore, increase the rate and force of contractions (via β-1 receptors).**
What is the effect of the sympathetic nervous system on the vasculature?	**Vasoconstriction (via α-1 receptors).** *Note: sympathetics do not vasoconstrict muscular arteries.*

What are the effects of increased sympathetic tone?	1. Increase heart rate (HR) and vasoconstriction of the vasculature, leading to increased cardiac work 2. Increase cardiac irritability, leading to arrhythmias 3. Coronary artery vasospasm 4. Discourage collateral circulation *Note: large lymphatic channels are under sympathetic control and therefore overactive sympathetics will impair lymphatic flow.*
Which lymphatic duct is responsible for draining the heart?	The right lymphatic duct. It also drains the right upper extremity, right side of the head, and both lungs.

CARDIOVASCULAR: CONGESTIVE HEART FAILURE

What is the pathologic process occurring in congestive heart failure (CHF)?	In CHF, the heart is unable to supply adequate blood flow to the tissues of the body.
What are common causes of CHF?	Hypertension (HTN), myocardial infarction (MI), and atherosclerosis are common etiologies.
How would HTN cause CHF?	HTN (or increased afterload) forces the heart to pump against a greater pressure. In response to the increased pressure, the heart muscle will hypertrophy and become weakened, therefore affecting contractility.
How would an MI cause CHF?	When an MI occurs, normal cardiac muscle is replaced by non-functional cardiac muscle (the tissue becomes hypokinetic). Again, this would weaken the myocardium and affect contractility.
How would atherosclerosis cause CHF?	Atherosclerosis, particularly of the coronary arteries, would decrease the amount of oxygen received by the heart and therefore decrease contractility.
Why is contractility so important in heart function?	Because a decrease in contractility will decrease the stroke volume (SV) and will therefore decrease the cardiac output (CO). *Note: $CO = HR \times SV$*
If a patient suffers from CHF, what medications should that patient receive for long-term management?	First-line treatments for long-term management of CHF are ACE inhibitors, β-blockers, digoxin, and spironolactone.

How can OMM be applied in the treatment of CHF?	**It works as adjunctive therapy in CHF patients because it normalizes lymphatics and autonomic nervous system (ANS). It accomplishes what pharmacologic therapy does without side effects or toxicity.**
How can OMM address the key treatment points of CHF?	**1. Decreasing excess fluid** **2. Increasing contractility.**
How can the treatment of lymphatics aid a patient with CHF?	Normalization of lymphatics aids in the correction of the fluid overload states.
What must always be done before initiating lymphatic techniques?	Open the thoracic inlet.
What two techniques facilitate respiration and therefore lymphatic flow?	• **Diaphragmatic lift** • **Treatment of any thoracic spine dysfunctions.**
What other simple lymphatic techniques can be used?	Lymphatic pumps (i.e., thoracic pump, pedal pump) will aid in restoring homeostasis.

CARDIOVASCULAR: MYOCARDIAL INFARCTION

What is the most common etiology of an MI?	MIs are frequently the result of an occlusive coronary thrombus.
What is the goal of therapy when treating an MI?	The immediate goal is reperfusion of the tissue affected by the thrombus.
What is management of a patient status post MI?	• Aspirin • Platelet aggregation inhibitors • Lipid lowering agents (statins, etc.) • β-blockers • ACE inhibitors • OMT
How can OMM address the key treatment points in post-MI patients?	**By normalizing ANS (↑ parasympathetics, ↓ sympathetics) and lymphatic system.**
What technique can be used to decrease sympathetic tone?	Rib-raising of ribs 1 to 6.
What techniques can be used to normalize parasympathetics?	• Condylar and OA decompression • Indirect treatment modalities to C_1, C_2, C_3 • Cranial techniques.

Why is lymphatic drainage important in a post-MI patient?	Lymphatic drainage will promote clearance of the damaged myocardium and effusion and therefore facilitate healing.
What techniques can be used to facilitate lymphatic drainage?	• Pectoral traction • Re-doming of the diaphragm • Any indirect, passive lymphatic treatment, this includes techniques such as the thoracic and pedal pump. *Remember: Lymphatics only work if the thoracic inlets are open first.*

CARDIOVASCULAR: HYPERTENSION

What is HTN?	HTN is an increased blood pressure that may result in organ damage and is characterized by a BP of greater than 140/90.
What causes HTN?	90% of HTN patients have no known etiology for their disorder.
HTN increases the risk for what health problems?	• Atherosclerotic cardiovascular disease • Stroke • CHF • Renal insufficiency
Malignant HTN (BP ≥ 210/140) can place patients at an increase for what serious medical problems?	• Encephalopathy • Intracranial hemorrhage • Unstable angina • MI • Left ventricular failure with concomitant pulmonary edema • Dissecting aorta • Renal failure.
What pharmacologic treatments can be used in HTN?	HTN is treated with diuretics, sympatholytics (β-blockers, α-blockers, or mixed adrenergic antagonists), calcium-channel blockers, ACE inhibitors, and direct-acting vasodilators.
How can OMM be applied in the treatment of HTN?	**It works as adjunctive therapy because it normalizes the ANS.**
How can OMM address the key treatment points of HTN?	By decreasing the sympathetic tone.

How does normalization of the sympathetics aid in treatment of HTN?	Decreasing sympathetic tone will: • decrease vascular resistance (via normalizing the body's hyperactive state of vasoconstriction). • decrease the heart rate.
What techniques can be used to normalize the sympathetics to the heart?	**Rib-raising and other paraspinal treatments should be performed along the entire sympathetic chain.**
What technique will directly affect catecholamine release?	T10 and T11 specifically address the adrenal glands, which may greatly contribute to HTN states because they increase epinephrine production. Chapman's points at this location will aid in normalizing adrenal function and therefore decrease the HR and force of contraction.

CARDIOVASCULAR: ARRHYTHMIAS

What is an arrhythmia?	It is any irregular heart rhythm, due to a defect in the electrical conduction system of the heart.
What are the three main subtypes of arrhythmias?	1. Premature complexes: these are more frequently from the ventricles and less often from the atria. 2. Tachyarrhythmias: have rates greater than 100 bpm and can be further divided into supraventricular tachycardias and ventricular tachycardias. 3. Bradyarrhythmias: have rates of less than 60 bpm.
What is the goal of management of patients with arrhythmias?	Rate and/or rhythm control.
How can OMM address the key treatment points in patients with arrhythmias?	**Treatment is dependent on the type of arrhythmia; however, the goals of treatment are fairly simple: if the heart is beating too fast, slow it down; if the heart is beating too slow, speed it up.**
What technique can be used in a tachyarrhythmic patient to normalize the sympathetic tone?	Rib-raising of ribs 1 to 6.
What techniques can be used in a bradyarrhythmia patient to normalize parasympathetic tone?	• Condylar and OA decompression • Indirect treatment modalities to C_1, C_2, C_3 • Cranial techniques

GASTROENTEROLOGY: ANATOMY AND OSTEOPATHIC PRINCIPLES

How does the parasympathetic nervous system affect the gastrointestinal (GI) system?	1. Contracts the muscles of the lumen. 2. Relaxes the muscle of the sphincter. 3. Increases secretion and motility.
Which three nerves and three ganglia are responsible for sympathetic innervation of most abdominal viscera.	1. Greater splanchnic nerve → celiac ganglion 2. Lesser splanchnic nerve → superior mesenteric ganglion 3. Least splanchnic nerve → inferior mesenteric ganglion.
What is the parasympathetic innervation of the GI tract?	**Vagus nerve to the foregut and midgut, sacral plexus (S2–S4) to hindgut.**
How does the sympathetic nervous system affect the GI system?	1. Relaxes the muscles of the lumen. 2. Contracts the muscle of the sphincter. 3. Decreases secretion and motility.
Which organs get sympathetic innervation from spinal cord region T5 to T9?	**Liver (T5–T9)** **Gallbladder (T5–T7, right)** **Stomach and proximal duodenum (T5–T9)** **Pancreas (T7)** **Spleen (T7, left)**
Which organs get sympathetic innervation from spinal cord region T10 to T12?	**Midgut including distal duodenum, jejunum, ileum, appendix, ascending colon and proximal $^2/_3$ transverse colon.**
Which organs get sympathetic innervation from spinal cord region T12 to L2?	**Hindgut including distal $^1/_3$ of transverse colon, descending colon, sigmoid colon, and rectum.**
What are the two significant intrinsic lymphatic pumps for abdominal lymphatics?	1. Peristalsis 2. Respiration.
What are three structural problems that can cause GI upset via vagal stimulation?	1. OA dysfunction 2. AA dysfunction 3. C_2 and C_3 dysfunction

What OMT technique can be used to treat a patient with ascites?	Lymphatic drainage
	1. First, the thoracic inlet must be opened
	2. Working on the thoracic and pelvic diaphragms (as well as the other diaphragms) is crucial to allow for effective lymphatic flow
	3. Finally, one can use the pedal pump, thoracic pump, or individual extremity lymphatic techniques to enhance lymphatic movement.

GASTROENTEROLOGY: GASTROESOPHAGEAL REFLUX DISEASE

What are the most common causes of gastroesophageal reflux disease (GERD)?	Most often, it is caused by transient lower esophageal sphincter (LES) relaxation. Other, less common reasons include decreased LES pressure and delayed gastric emptying.
What risk factors are associated with GERD?	1. Ingestion of alcohol, fat, chocolate, or mints and smoking all decrease LES pressure
	2. Hiatal hernia alters the GE junction
	3. Intra-abdominal pressure increase secondary to obesity
	4. Medications that reduce LES pressure (benzodiazepines, narcotics, calcium-channel blockers, anticholinergics).
What are the non-pharmacologic treatments for GERD?	Elevate head, lose weight, quit smoking, decrease caffeine and alcohol intake, avoid foods and medications that lower LES pressure, avoid meals within 2 hours of lying down, and frequent small high-protein meals.
What are the pharmacologic treatments for GERD?	H2 receptor antagonists, prokinetics, and proton pump inhibitors, antacids.
What are the complications of GERD?	Esophageal ulceration, peptic stricture, Barrett's esophagus, adenocarcinoma, bleeding, pulmonary problems, and non-cardiac chest pain.
Which ANS can be targeted using OMT to help treat GERD?	Since the LES is relaxed, by normalizing the parasympathetic tone, sphincter tone can be increased.
Addressing what area of the body is most effective in the management GERD?	**Vagal trunks supply the abdominal part of the esophagus; thus, treating the OA is effective. Also, as the LES is surrounded by the diaphragm, diaphragmatic dysfunction may decrease LES competency and must be addressed.**

By normalizing the parasympathetic nervous system, which other physiologic process is also controlled in the treatment of GERD?

The secretion of acid in the stomach by the parietal cells is largely controlled by the vagus. Treatment of the OA can help reduce acid production, which helps decrease reflux (also helpful in patients with peptic ulcer disease).

GASTROENTEROLOGY: CHOLECYSTITIS

What is acute cholecystitis and what is the most common cause?

Inflammation of the gallbladder, usually secondary to biliary tract obstruction by a stone.

What are the three types of gallstones?

1. Cholesterol gallstones
2. Pigment gallstones
3. Mixed gallstones.

What are the risk factors for cholesterol gallstones and subsequent cholecystitis?

1. **F**at
2. **F**emale
3. **F**ertile
4. **F**orty
5. **F**latulent.

 ***Memory Aid:* F**ive **F**s

Continued gallbladder dysfunction due to gallstones will result in segmental facilitation of which region?

T5 to T7 on the right.

Referred pain to what extremity region is commonly seen in cholecystitis?

Right shoulder, irritation of the diaphragm is thought to cause phrenic nerve (C3–C5) inflammation radiating to the shoulder.

How can OMT be applied in the treatment of cholecystitis?

Treat the somatic dysfunctions of the shoulder and address C3–C5 (phrenic n.). Treat the OA to normalize parasympathetics via the vagus n., thus helping with secretions. Finally, normalize sympathetic innervation by addressing thoracic facilitations.

GASTROENTEROLOGY: IRRITABLE BOWEL SYNDROME

What is irritable bowel syndrome (IBS)?

Motility disorder involving the entire GI tract; causes recurring upper and lower GI symptoms. Accounting for up to 50% of patients referred to a gastroenterologist.

What are the signs and symptoms of IBS?

Abdominal pain, diarrhea, constipation, alternating constipation and diarrhea, gas, bloating, incomplete evacuation, tenesmus, rectal pain, or mucus in the stool.

What is the epidemiology of IBS?	2:1 female:male ratio and higher in Caucasians.
How is IBS diagnosed?	It is a diagnosis of exclusion in a healthy appearing individual with a normal examination, yet present with GI symptoms.
What is the classical treatment for IBS?	1. Emotional support and stress reduction 2. Diet and fiber therapy 3. Medications: antispasmodics, laxatives, anti-diarrhea, antidepressants 4. OMT.
How can IBS be treated using OMT?	**Treatment begins with opening up the abdominal and pelvic diaphragms followed by normalizing autonomic tone (sympathetic chain, cranium, OA, sacral plexus). The intense fluctuations that accompany this disease cause muscle tension, including tension to the diaphragms. Lymphatic techniques are also significant as there is also an inflammatory component to IBS.**

GASTROENTEROLOGY: INFLAMMATORY BOWEL DISEASE

What are the forms of inflammatory bowel disease?	Crohn's disease (CD) and ulcerative colitis (UC). They are characterized by chronic bowel inflammation.
Which form of IBD is limited to the colon?	UC. CD can occur anywhere from the mouth to the anus, with rectal sparing. *Memory Aid:* <u>Col</u>on—Ulcerative <u>Col</u>itis.
Which form of IBD more commonly presents with bleeding and is associated with greater risk of carcinoma?	UC
What are the extra-intestinal manifestations of IBD and in which disease are they most often encountered?	1. **Primary sclerosing cholangitis: UC** 2. **Large joint arthritis: UC and CD** 3. **Pyoderma gangrenosum: UC and CD** 4. **Uveitis: UC and CD** 5. **Ankylosing spondylitis: CD** 6. **Sacroiliitis: CD** 7. **Erythema nodosum: CD** 8. **Episcleritis: CD** 9. **Aphthous ulcers: CD**

What is the medical treatment for CD?	Treatment depends on the severity of inflammation and the involved region. Medications include 5-ASA derivatives, corticosteroids, antibiotics, immunosuppressives, and OMT.
What are the most common complications of UC?	1. Toxic megacolon 2. Colonic perforation 3. Colon cancer.
How can IBD be treated using OMT?	**Treatment begins with opening up the abdominal and pelvic diaphragms followed by normalizing autonomic tone (sympathetic chain, cranium, OA, sacral plexus). The intense fluctuations that accompany this disease cause muscle tension, including tension to the diaphragms. Lymphatic techniques will also aid in lowering symptoms and disease progression.**

NEPHROLOGY

What is the autonomic innervation to the kidneys?	**Sympathetic innervation: T10 to T11** **Parasympathetic innervation: Vagus n. (limited).**

What is the autonomic innervation to the ureters?	**Upper ureter (or abdominal section):**
	
	    Sympathetics — T10 through T11/T12
	
	    Parasympathetic — Vagus n.
	
	Lower ureter (or pelvic section):
	
	    Sympathetics — T12/L1 through L2
	
	    Parasympathetics — S2 through S4.

What are the major roles of the ANS on the ureter?	The ANS affects peristalsis of the ureter.
What muscular findings are found with kidney and ureter pathology?	The quadratus lumborum and psoas mm. are often rigid or in spasm with kidney or ureter disease. These can be treated with lumbar, innominate, or hip muscle energy.
Where are the Chapman's points that correspond to the kidney?	**Anterior Chapman points are located one-inch superior and one-inch lateral to the umbilicus. Posterior Chapman points are located between the spinous process and transverse process of T_{12} and L_1.**
What is the major stimulus that results in ureteral somatic dysfunctions?	Somatic manifestations from the ureters occur most commonly from dilation of the ureter from a distal obstruction.

What are the common somatic dysfunctions found with ureteral pathology?	Upper ureter: Flank pain and muscular rigidity in the dermatomes of T11 through T12 (above anterior superior iliac spine and extending medially to the rectus femoris). Middle ureter: Pain can be observed in dermatomes T12 and L1 (along the inguinal ligament up to the rectus femoris). Lower ureter: Pain follows dermatomes L1 and L2 (suprapubic and below the labia/scrotum).

RHEUMATOLOGY

Describe osteoarthritis.	A disorder in which joint articular cartilage deteriorates and is replaced by new bone formation.
What joints are commonly affected in osteoarthritis?	**Distal interphalangeal (DIP) > proximal interphalangeal (PIP) > first metacarpophalangeal > knees > hips > metatarsophalangeal**
What are common signs and symptoms of osteoarthritis?	**Pain, morning stiffness (<30 minutes), tenderness, decreased and often painful range of motion of joints, joint enlargement (swelling), Heberden's nodes (at DIP joint), Bouchard's nodes (at PIP joint), and osteophytes.**
Describe rheumatoid arthritis (RA).	It is a systemic chronic inflammatory disease of unknown etiology that involves many symmetric joints. Granulation tissue develops in the joint spaces and erodes the cartilage and bone. Rheumatoid factor is commonly positive in the serum, which tends to correlate with more severe disease. Patients with this disorder have an increased prevalence of HLA-DR4.
What joints are commonly involved in RA?	**PIP > metacarpophalangeal > wrist > knees > ankles**
What are common signs and symptoms of RA?	**Malaise, anorexia, fatigue, hypertrophy of synovial tissue, morning stiffness ≥1 hour, joint pain, painless rheumatic nodules, cervical spine instability due to erosion of the bone. Systemic manifestations include pleuritis, vasculitis, and pulmonary nodules.**
What osteopathic findings and treatments should be considered in patients with arthritis?	Hypersympathetic tone leads to decreased blood and lymphatic flow at joints. Hypersympathetic tone can be treated with rib-raising. Decreased blood and lymphatic flow can be treated with articulatory and lymphatic techniques. Fascial restrictions and tenderpoints should also be treated.

What role does hypersympathetic tone play in RA?	Hypersympathetics can constrict the blood vessels and lymphatics that supply joints thus decreasing oxygen delivery and metabolite removal. It can also heighten a patient's pain sensitivity, increase muscle spasm and decrease range of motion.
What osteopathic treatment is contraindicated in RA?	**Cervical HVLA, because of weakened cruciate ligaments (especially C$_2$).**
How can a patient actively aid in their treatment?	Weight loss to decrease stress on joints, stretching and exercise to increase range of motion and improve blood and lymphatic flow.
Describe scleroderma.	It is a connective tissue disease resulting in systemic fibrosis, usually starting with the skin but also affecting many organs.
What are the two major classifications of scleroderma? Which is more likely to be fatal?	Diffuse and limited scleroderma. Diffuse scleroderma is more likely to be fatal.
What are the signs and symptoms of scleroderma?	Tightening of the skin, Raynaud's phenomenon, dysphagia, esophageal strictures, telangiectasias, calcifications, renal artery fibrosis, and pulmonary hypertension.
What is limited scleroderma?	It is another name for **CREST** syndrome, which consists of **C**alcinosis, **R**aynaud's phenomenon, **E**sophageal dysmotility, **S**clerodactyly, and **T**elangiectasias. The skin involvement is generally limited to the hands and sometimes the face/neck. Digital ulcers and lung fibrosis are also common.
What osteopathic treatments for Raynaud's phenomenon can be effective?	Treatment focuses on signs such as endothelial fibrosis and vasoconstriction. Normalizing sympathetic tone to decrease vasoconstriction and improve blood supply. Treating all diaphragms starting with the thoracic inlet and progressing distally along the upper extremity is also effective.
What is the osteopathic treatment for esophageal dysmotility?	**Treat parasympathetics (OA and AA) to ↑ peristalsis and normalize sympathetics (T1 to T8).**

ENDOCRINOLOGY: ANATOMY AND OSTEOPATHIC PRINCIPLES

What is the function of the hypothalamus and pituitary gland?	The hypothalamus and pituitary function as a major control center for the internal environment and its response to external stimuli.
How does the primary respiratory mechanism influence the hypothalamus?	**Reduction of the rate and amplitude of the primary respiratory mechanism will reduce the fluctuations in CSF, which is a major signaling device for the hypothalamus. Also, movement of the sphenoid bone and the sphenobasilar junction contributes to the circulation of the hypothalamic pituitary portal system.**
How are the hypothalamus and pituitary gland treated?	Directly by cranial treatments and indirectly via spinal manipulation of somatic dysfunctions, somatovisceral reflexes, and lymphatic techniques.
What is the most important region to focus on while attempting to treat the hypothalamus/pituitary gland?	**The sphenobasilar junction due to its proximity.**

ENDOCRINOLOGY: THYROID DISEASE

What are the autonomics to the thyroid gland?	Sympathetic innervation of T1 to T4 causes vasoconstriction of the blood supply to the gland. Parasympathetic innervation is delivered via the vagus n.
What are the main forms of thyroid hormones?	Thyroxine (T_4) made only in the thyroid. Triiodothyronine (T_3) is made mostly from peripheral conversion of T_4 to T_3.
What produces thyroid-stimulating hormone (TSH)?	The anterior pituitary gland synthesizes and releases TSH in response to thyrotropin-releasing hormone (TRH).
What are common somatic findings associated with thyroid dysfunction?	1. **OA, AA, C_3 and T_1 to T_4 dysfunction** 2. **Chapman's points: intercostals between ribs 2 and 3, close to sternum and middle of transverse process of T_2.**
What are the signs and symptoms of hyperthyroidism?	Warm, moist, diaphoretic skin; clubbing of fingers/toes, infiltrative ophthalmopathy, lid tremor/lag, sinus tachycardia, dyspnea, resting tremor.

What is the medical treatment of hyperthyroidism?	1. Anti-thyroid medications: PTU and methimazole 2. Radiation 3. Radioactive iodine.
How can OMT be used to treat hyperthyroidism?	Treat the symptoms that were mentioned above, normalize sympathetics along the entire sympathetic chain to help with tachycardia and diaphoresis. Enhance lung function via doming of the diaphragm and rib raising. Cranial treatments will help with imbalance caused by the pituitary gland.
What is hypothyroidism?	Clinical syndrome due to the deficiency of thyroid hormones.
What are the symptoms of hypothyroidism?	Non-pitting edema, dry hair, temporal thinning of brows, fatigue, constipation, cold intolerance, decreased appetite, weight gain, depression.
What is the medical treatment of hypothyroidism?	Levothyroxine (T_4) most often used.
How can OMT be used to treat hypothyroidism?	Treat the symptoms that were mentioned above, normalize sympathetics while working on parasympathetics to help with constipation. Lymphatic techniques will decrease edema. Cranial treatments will help with imbalance caused by the pituitary gland.
What role does OMT of the lymphatics play in autoimmune thyroid disease?	Lymphatic techniques are crucial in presenting antibodies responsible for thyroid instability to the immune system.

ENDOCRINOLOGY: DIABETES MELLITUS

What is diabetes mellitus (DM)?	Disorder that is characterized by either absolute insulin deficiency or insulin resistance, resulting in hyperglycemia.
What is type I DM?	Autoimmune destruction of the pancreatic islet beta cells resulting in insulin deficiency, requiring exogenous insulin.
What is type II DM?	A combination of insulin resistance and delayed insulin secretion after a glucose challenge, most often not requiring exogenous insulin.

How can OMT be used to treat DM?	Normalize autonomics to the adrenal glands (T10–T11) using the ribs and thoracic vertebrae.
	Note: One theory states that because type I DM may be due to an autoimmune process, treating the lymphatics can increase presentation of these autoimmune processes to the immune system.

ENDOCRINOLOGY: ADDISON'S DISEASE

What is Addison's disease?	Addison's disease is hypoaldosteronism and hypocortisolism due to dysfunction or destruction of the adrenal cortices.
What is the most common cause of Addison's disease?	Autoimmune (80%).
What is the clinical presentation of Addison's disease?	Weakness, anorexia, weight loss, abdominal pain, nausea/vomiting, diarrhea, flushing, hypotension, mucosal hyperpigmentation.
What lab findings are associated with Addison's disease?	Decreased: Na^+, cortisol, aldosterone, androgens Increased: K^+, Ca^{2+}, BUN
How is Addison's disease treated medically?	Treatment is with hydrocortisone or fludrocortisone.

ENDOCRINOLOGY: CUSHING'S SYNDROME

What is Cushing's syndrome?	Primary or secondary hypercortisolism
What is the most common cause of Cushing's syndrome?	Iatrogenic from long-term use of glucocorticoids for the treatment of asthma and arthritis
What is the clinical presentation of Cushing's syndrome?	Central obesity ("moon face," "buffalo hump"), hirsutism, and cutaneous striae.
Where are facilitations resulting from adrenal pathology found?	T_{10}–T_{11}
Where are Chapman's points located corresponding to the adrenal glands?	**Anterior Chapman's points for the adrenal glands are approximately 2 inches superior and one-inch lateral of the umbilicus. Posterior Chapman's point corresponding to the adrenal glands is on the spinous process of T_{11}.**

221

CHAPTER

16 PEDIATRICS

BIRTHING ISSUES

When do the anterior and posterior fontanelles close?	**Anterior fontanelle: 1–2 years old** **Posterior fontanelle: 2 months of age**
Which bone is most commonly susceptible to somatic dysfunction (SD) from the birthing process?	The occiput. At birth, it is composed of four parts. It is exposed to multiple and complex forces during the birthing process.
What everyday activities of an infant will correct most cranial SD that are acquired from birthing process?	Sucking and crying. *Note: Cranial osteopathy is indicated in cases of inappropriate suckling/nursing.*
What nerve entrapments can be seen with occipital condylar compression?	**CN IX, CN X, CN XI at the jugular foramen and CN XII at the hypoglossal foramen. These can manifest as problems with feeding in the newborn.**
The use of forceps during delivery can result in injury of what nerve?	**Facial nerve (CN VII) at the stylomastoid foramen because the developing mastoid process is unable to protect the stylomastoid foramen laterally.**
What is the most commonly fractured bone during delivery?	**Clavicle.**
What factors predispose neonates to clavicle fractures during parturition?	Large for gestational age and shoulder dystocia.
What are common physical exam findings with clavicle fractures in neonates?	Asymmetric Moro reflex and crepitus over fracture.
How are clavicle fractures treated?	Immobilization for 3 to 4 weeks, followed by the Spencer technique and counterstrain to regain any lost range of motion.
What is the pathophysiology of meconium aspiration?	The meconium obstructs the alveoli leading to air-trapping and hyperinflation; pneumothorax may occur.
What is the role of OMT in meconium aspiration?	Improve lymphatics and correction of any SD that could contribute to airway hyperactivity and hyperinflation.

NEONATOLOGY

What is another name for neonatal respiratory distress syndrome (NRDS)?	Hyaline membrane disease due to the deposition of fibrin and protein into alveolar spaces secondary to inflammation and surfactant deficiency. This causes obstruction of gas exchange.
What are common signs of surfactant deficiency?	Grunting, nasal flaring, sternal/intercostal retractions, and tachypnea.
What are the common therapeutic approaches to NRDS?	**Mechanical ventilation with positive end-expiratory pressure (PEEP), exogenous surfactant, maintenance of pH and BP, OMT.**
What is the role of OMT in patients with NRDS?	Improving lymphatic drainage decreases surface tension, which in turn decreases the need for PEEP. Treatment of ribs and vertebrae decreases chest wall resistance.
What is transient tachypnea of the newborn?	Tachypnea and cyanosis due to the delay of removal of intrapulmonary fluid. It usually resolves in 48 hours and is more common in newborns delivered by C-section due to compression of lungs.
What somatic dysfunctions are associated with transient tachypnea of the newborn?	Restriction of normal newborn respiratory mechanics usually due to SD at thoracolumbar and pelvic areas and restrictions of quadratus lumborum and scalene muscles.
What is the role of OMT in transient tachypnea of the newborn?	Correcting the SD improves the respiratory mechanics. The intrapulmonary fluids decrease, leading to earlier resolution of the tachypnea.

RESPIRATORY

What is croup?	Viral infection that causes inflammation and edema of the subglottic area.
What is the classic presentation of croup?	**A child who had cold symptoms for several days followed by a barking cough.**
What is the classical radiologic finding for croup?	**"Steeple" sign on AP neck x-ray.**

What is the osteopathic approach to a patient with croup?	Because the inflammation and edema are caused by vasodilation, stimulation of sympathetics at T1–T6 causes vasoconstriction (using the same mechanism as giving racemic epinephrine). Normalizing the parasympathetics to the trachea may also be of benefit in the case of heightened parasympathetic nervous system tone.
What is bronchiolitis?	An acute viral infection of the lower respiratory tract; usually in children younger than 2 years old.
What areas should be assessed for SD in a patient with bronchiolitis?	**Cervical region—C_3 to C_5 (phrenic nerve); OA and AA (vagus nerve).**
	Rib cage—Decreases work of breathing and enhances lymphatic drainage.
	Rib-raising: T_1–T_6—Normalize sympathetics to the airways.
	Thoracic diaphragm—Improves tidal volume.
	Sacrum dura has attachments at foramen magnum, C_2, C_3, and S_2, which can alter parasympathetics to the lungs.
	Temporal bones—Internal rotation restriction leads to shallow breathing.

JUVENILE RHEUMATOID ARTHRITIS

What is juvenile rheumatoid arthritis (JRA)?	Chronic non-suppurative inflammation of the synovium and joint effusion followed by bony destruction.
What is the classical presentation of JRA?	**Morning stiffness, uveitis, joint pain that is worse in morning and improves throughout the day, swelling, and decreased range of motion.**
What is the osteopathic approach to a patient with JRA?	Treatment of lymphatics, sympathetics, and parasympathetics to maximize circulation to the joints and techniques to improve function and range of motion.
What OMM technique should be avoided in a patient with JRA?	**HVLA**

ORTHOPEDICS

At what age is the cervical lordosis present?	At birth. Increases as the infant becomes able to lift head.
At what age does the thoracic kyphosis develop?	Age 8–9 months when infant starts to sit upright.
At what age does the lumbar lordosis develop?	13 months to 5 years as the toddler begins to crawl and progresses with walking.
What is scoliosis?	An abnormal curvature of the spine in the coronal and/or sagittal planes. Adams test and Cobb method may be used for scoliosis screening and classification, respectively. *See Chapter 5: Thoracic Spine—Clinical Anatomy and Special Tests for more information on scoliosis and testing.*
What is the difference between a structural and functional curve?	**Structural: fixed and inflexible; does not correct with sidebending to opposite side.** **Functional: flexible and corrects with sidebending to opposite side.**
What is the treatment of scoliosis?	Mild: physical therapy and OMT. Moderate: above treatments plus spinal orthotics. Severe: surgery if respiratory compromise.
What are the two types of short leg discrepancies?	Anatomic (congenital): leg is shorter. Functional: leg appears shorter.
What dysfunctions are associated with short leg syndrome?	• Sacral base is lower on side of short leg. • Anterior innominate rotation on contralateral side to short leg. • Posterior innominate rotation on ipsilateral side of short leg. • Lumbar spine sidebends away and rotates toward side of short leg.
What is the treatment of short leg syndrome (anatomic and functional)?	**OMT to correct SD as much as possible, then a heel lift if the difference in femoral head heights is >5 mm on a postural x-ray.**

What are common signs used to diagnose developmental dysplasia of the hip?

Barlow test: while stabilizing pelvis with one hand, the opposite hip is flexed and adducted. The dislocation can be felt.

Ortolani's test: hip is flexed and abducted. The femoral head is placed back into acetabulum and a click may be felt.

Galezzi's sign: with infant supine and knees and hips flexed, the knee will be lower on side of dislocation.

What is the best test for developmental dysplasia of the hip in newborns?

Ultrasound. It shows the unossified cartilaginous femoral head and acetabulum.

What is nursemaid's elbow?

Subluxation of the radial head after sudden longitudinal traction on the arm usually in an extended and pronated position.

How is nursemaid's elbow treated?

By taking the arm from a pronated extended position to a supinated flexed position while putting pressure over radial head in an anterior direction.

Chapter 17

OBSTETRICS AND GYNECOLOGY

PREGNANCY

In the osteopathic structural exam, what typical cranial findings are important to assess in the pregnant patient?

1. Cranial rhythmic impulse (CRI) (crucial to maintenance of homeostasis)
2. Strain patterns (affects sacral motion, important in labor and delivery)
3. Occipito-atlantal (OA) dysfunction (affects parasympathetics to the abdominal viscera via the vagus)
4. OM suture (compression affects vagal tone).

In the osteopathic structural exam, what typical cervical vertebral findings are important to assess in the pregnant patient?

1. C_2 dysfunction (affects vagal/parasympathetics to the abdominal viscera);
2. C_{2-5} (facilitation at these segments affects phrenic n. innervation of the abdominal diaphragm).

In the osteopathic structural exam, what typical thoracic findings are important to assess in the pregnant patient?

1. Increased kyphosis
2. Scoliosis
3. T_{4-7} dysfunction (associated with breast tenderness)
4. Thoracic inlet (important consideration in lymphatic return)
5. Rib excursion.

What typical lumbar findings are important to assess in the pregnant patient?

1. Increased lordosis
2. Paraspinal muscle spasm (facilitation to/from pelvic viscera)
3. Lumbosacral junction restriction
4. Tension in iliolumbar ligament.

What typical sacral findings are important to assess in the pregnant patient?

1. Sacral shears/torsions
2. Sacral respiratory motion
3. Sacral/cranial motion.

What typical ilial findings are important to assess in the pregnant patient?

Ilial rotation/shears.

What diaphragmatic restrictions are important to assess in the pregnant patient?	1. Cranial (falx and tentorium cerebelli) 2. Thoracic inlet 3. Thoracoabdominal 4. Pelvic.
What lower extremity findings are important to assess in the pregnant patient?	1. Leg length (length discrepancy associated with pelvic and sacral dysfunction, and round ligament strain) 2. Edema.
What are the stages of pregnancy as they relate to osteopathic considerations?	1. Structural stage 2. Congestive stage 3. Preparatory stage 4. Labor and delivery 5. Recovery and maintenance stage.
Define the structural stage of pregnancy.	The first week to the 28th week of pregnancy. During this stage, osteopathic concerns center around changes in the musculoskeletal system as a result of the pregnancy.
What somatic dysfunctions are commonly found in the structural stage of pregnancy?	1. Anterior pelvis (pelvis rocks forward) 2. Sacral somatic dysfunction (SD) (sacral shears are common) 3. Lumbar SD (increased lordosis) 4. Thoracic SD (increased kyphosis, T_4–T_7 SD associated with breast tenderness) 5. Cervical SD (increased cervical lordosis recurrent C_2 SD/occipital strain).
What osteopathic treatments may be beneficial in the structural stage of pregnancy?	1. No modality of osteopathic treatment is contraindicated in the structural stage of pregnancy. 2. Rib raising to normalize sympathetic tone. 3. Sacral rock improves parasympathetic influences (S_2–S_4), which may decrease the incidence of hyperemesis gravidarum/"morning sickness". 4. OM suture decompression normalizes vagal tone, decreasing incidence of nausea/vomiting, reflux, and constipation.
Define the congestive stage of pregnancy.	The 28th through 36th weeks of pregnancy. During this stage of pregnancy, osteopathic concerns center around changes in fluid homeostasis as a result of the pregnancy. This is a state of increased fluids with diminished mechanisms to remove them.

What somatic dysfunctions are commonly found in the congestive stage of pregnancy?	1. Fascial strains at the thoracic inlet 2. Diaphragmatic restrictions (pelvic and thoracoabdominal diaphragms, falx, and tentorium cerebelli) 3. Lumbar strain and SD 4. Pelvic and sacral SD 5. Rib SD 6. Lower extremity edema.
What osteopathic treatments may be beneficial in the congestive stage of pregnancy?	1. No modality of osteopathic treatment is contraindicated in the congestive stage of pregnancy; however, HVLA should be used with caution 2. Thoracic inlet release 3. Lymphatic drainage/pump 4. Compression of the fourth ventricle (CV_4) 5. Pectoral lift 6. Thoracoabdominal diaphragmatic doming 7. Pelvic diaphragm release.
Define the preparatory stage of pregnancy.	The 36th week through delivery. During this stage of pregnancy, osteopathic concerns center around maintaining good structural balance, maintenance of lymphatic flow, and effective craniosacral mechanism.
What somatic dysfunctions are commonly found in the preparatory stage of pregnancy?	1. Sacral base anterior 2. Increased lumbar strain 3. Increased pelvic diaphragm restriction.
What osteopathic treatments may be beneficial in the preparatory stage of pregnancy?	1. **HVLA is contraindicated in the preparatory stage of pregnancy in the pelvis and lumbar spine because of the effects of relaxin hormone on the ligaments** 2. **Sacral rock** 3. **CV_4** 4. **Lumbosacral (LS) joint release** 5. **Pelvic diaphragm release.**
Define the labor and delivery stage of pregnancy.	The onset of labor through delivery. During this stage of pregnancy, osteopathic concerns center around good sacral/pelvic motion and effective uterine contractions.

What somatic dysfunction is of special concern in the labor and delivery stage of pregnancy?	Sacral restrictions/SD.
What are the normal motions of the sacrum in labor and delivery?	1. Sacral extension (counternutation) occurs during engagement 2. Sacral flexion (nutation) occurs during descent and delivery.
What other SDs are of special concern in the labor and delivery stage of pregnancy?	1. Decreased amplitude of the CRI 2. Adducted pubic dysfunction.
What osteopathic treatments may be beneficial in the labor and delivery stage of pregnancy?	1. CV_4 and sacral rock to stimulate/augment uterine contractions 2. Sacral rock to improve sacral motion 3. Pelvic diaphragm release may improve descent 4. Muscle energy (ME) to treat adducted pubic dysfunction and facilitate vaginal delivery.
Define the recovery and maintenance stage of pregnancy.	Delivery through 6 weeks postpartum. During this stage of pregnancy, osteopathic concerns center around correcting sacral motion, decreasing lymphatic congestion, and restoring proper functional position of the junctions.
What SDs are of special concern in the recovery and maintenance stage of pregnancy?	1. **Sacral flexion (nutation)** 2. **Pelvic diaphragm restriction** 3. **Sacroiliac dysfunction resulting from increased elasticity of pelvic ligaments.**
What osteopathic treatments may be beneficial in the recovery and maintenance stage of pregnancy?	1. Sacral rock to release sacral flexion (anterior sacral base, nutation) 2. CV_4 to restore homeostasis of body fluids, decreases the incidence of post-partum depression by increasing the CRI 3. A lymphatic pump decreases fluid congestion reducing breast congestion.
What are the contraindications to osteopathic treatment in pregnancy?	1. Undiagnosed vaginal bleeding 2. Threatened or incomplete abortion 3. Ectopic pregnancy 4. Placenta previa 5. Placental abruption 6. Pre-term/premature rupture of membranes 7. Prolapsed umbilical cord 8. Eclampsia and severe preeclampsia.

What techniques can be used to balance autonomic tone?	1. Rib raising (decrease sympathetic tone) 2. Treating somatic dysfunction at: OM suture, OA, atlanto-axial, C_2 (to improve vagal tone).
What techniques can be used to promote fluid homeostasis?	1. Release of fascial contractures/restrictions 2. Lymphatic pumps 3. Thoracic inlet, thoracoabdominal and pelvic diaphragm release.
What conditions of pregnancy can be treated by improving fluid homeostasis?	1. Hypertension 2. Hyperemesis/nausea/vomiting, reflux, and constipation 3. Hemorrhoids.
What is the osteopathic treatment of carpal tunnel syndrome in pregnancy?	1. Decrease fluid congestion by improving lymphatic flow (lymphatic pumps) 2. Release thoracic inlet fascial restrictions 3. Rib raising to normalize upper extremity sympathetic innervation (T1 or T2 through T8) 4. Myofascial release of the flexor retinaculum.
What is the osteopathic treatment of round ligament pain in pregnancy?	**1. Correct posterior innominate rotation that may stretch the ipsilateral round ligament** **2. Treat leg length discrepancy that may strain the round ligament.**

PELVIC PAIN

What is a common somatic manifestation of pelvic visceral dysfunction?	Low back pain.
What muscle may cause gynecologic dysfunction due to its proximity to vascular, neural, and lymphatic elements of the reproductive organs?	Psoas muscle.
At what spinal level might somatic dysfunction be found on structural exam for the pelvic viscera?	
Ovaries	T_{10-11}
Uterus	T_{10}–L_2
Fallopian tubes	T_{11}–T_{12}
Vagina	T_{10}–L_2
Cervix	S_2–S_4
What major restriction plays a role in producing symptoms associated with pelvic pain?	Pelvic diaphragm restriction.

List characteristic somatic dysfunctions associated with pelvic pain.	1. Iliacus m. tenderpoint (iliac fossa to the tendon of psoas)
	2. Quadratus lumborum m. spasm
	3. Chapman's reflex points
	4. Sacral somatic dysfunction
	5. Lower thoracic and lumbar somatic dysfunction
	6. Thoracoabdominal diaphragm restrictions
	7. Ligamentous strains (e.g., iliolumbar ligament, uterosacral ligament, etc.).

Where are the Chapman's reflex points for the pelvic viscera?

Uterus	Iliotibial band, anterior portion of the pubic bone, and transverse process of L_5
Ovaries	Ramus of the pubic bone and transverse process of T_{10}
Fallopian tubes	Posterior superior iliac spine
Vagina	Sacral base and medial aspect of posterior thigh.
	See Figure 1.1 in Chapman's Reflex Points.

What osteopathic treatments may be beneficial in the treatment of pelvic congestion associated with pelvic pain?	1. Pelvic and thoracoabdominal diaphragm release
	2. Lymphatic pumps
	3. Rib raising (to normalize sympathetic tone to the lymphatics)
	4. Sacral rocking (to normalize parasympathetic tone).

What osteopathic techniques may be beneficial in the treatment of viscerosomatic reflexes associated with pelvic pain?	ME, facilitated positional release, HVLA, or counterstrain may be used to treat somatic dysfunction found at the involved spinal level.

What osteopathic techniques may be beneficial in the treatment of ligamentous strains associated with pelvic pain?	**Ligamentous articular strain/balanced ligamentous tension.**

What osteopathic techniques may be beneficial in treating muscle spasm associated with pelvic pain (psoas or quadratus lumborum m. spasm)?	Inhibition and ME.

OSTEOPATHIC PRINCIPLES

How can the cranial rhythmic impulse (CRI) be evaluated?	By assessing the cranial and sacral motion.
How does CRI change in the psychiatric patient?	**CRI is generally decreased.**
How can OMT be used in healing psychiatric patients?	1. Normalize sympathetics (calming effect) 2. Increasing CRI.
What is another name for the somato-emotional release experienced by patients during OMT?	**Tissue memory.**
What regions should osteopathic treatment focus on in patients after electroconvulsive therapy?	Techniques directed to the cranial, sacral, and pelvic areas.
Where are somatic dysfunctions found in psychiatric patients?	**Sympathetic hyperstimulation most commonly manifests at the levels of C_2, T_4–T_6, and the sacrum (S_2).**

CONTRAINDICATIONS

What are the contraindications to OMT in psychiatric patients?	Some osteopathic techniques can appear physically threatening and are therefore a relative contraindication in sexually abused patients, delusional schizophrenics, and those suffering from active hallucinations.
Osteopathic manipulation to what regions should be limited in sexually abused patients?	Sacrum and pelvis and other sexually sensitive areas such as middle ribs or sternum should be avoided.

19 GENERAL SURGERY

POSTOPERATIVE FEVER

What are the typical patterns of postoperative fever?

1. <u>W</u>ind: Pulmonary complications, usually days 1–3.
   a. Atelectasis
   b. Pneumonia

2. <u>W</u>ater: Urinary tract infection, usually days 3–5, usually after bladder catheterization.

3. <u>W</u>ound infections: Cause fever beginning days 5–8. Only streptococcal and clostridial wound infections cause earlier fever.

4. <u>W</u>alk: Venous complications, days 7–10.
   a. Deep venous thrombosis
   b. Pulmonary embolism
   c. Intravenous catheter infections

5. <u>W</u>onder drugs: Drug fever from anesthetics and antibiotics being used empirically, highly variable, could occur any day.

6. <u>W</u>omb: In a pregnant patient, remain alert for postpartum endometritis and chorioamnionitis.

 Memory Aid: 6 <u>W</u>s.

How can atelectasis be treated?

Remove diaphragmatic, thoracic, rib, and lumbar dysfunctions. Airflow has to be improved to treat atelectasis (encourage incentive spirometry). The thoracic lymphatic pump has been effective in the prevention of atelectasis in the postoperative period.

What is the thoracic lymphatic pump?

The thoracic lymphatic pump is a ventilator assist technique that uses passive and active rib excursion. Patients treated with the thoracic lymphatic pump had an earlier recovery and faster return to preoperative values for both the forced vital capacity and FEV_1.

Does an abscess cause facilitation?

Most of the time an abscess does not cause facilitation in the spine because it is walled off by epithelium.

How can one improve the immune response of the patient?	Correction of somatic dysfunction at the transition zones (i.e., cervicothoracic/thoracolumbar/ lumbosacral junctions), improve lymphatic fluid flow by diaphragmatic motion in both the abdominal and pelvic diaphragms, respectively. Depending on the condition of the patient, one may also perform a thoracic, pedal or splenic pump.

POSTOPERATIVE ILEUS

What is paralytic ileus (A.K.A. postoperative ileus)?	**A functional obstruction of the small bowel that occurs in patients following abdominal surgery and is caused by a combination of neural, humoral, and metabolic factors. It can also occur with inflammatory processes, such as peritonitis, retroperitoneal hemorrhage, pancreatitis, spinal injury, electrolytes, and medications.**
What are the typical signs of ileus?	Lack of bowel sounds and inability to pass flatus or stool.
What is the order of return of motility following abdominal surgery?	1. Small intestine 2. Stomach 3. Colon.
What is the physiologic cause of ileus?	A hypersympathetic response that slows gastrointestinal propulsion and constricts various sphincters.
How can ileus be treated?	**Nothing by mouth, nasogastric tube, intravenous fluids with electrolyte replacement as needed and osteopathic manipulation to decrease hypersympathetic input.**
Which levels of the spinal cord correspond to the small intestines?	**Sympathetic: T10 through T11 or T12** **Parasympathetic: Vagus n. (CN X)**
What osteopathic techniques can be used to decrease sympathetic drive in the treatment of paralytic ileus?	Balance ligamentous tension, rib raising, articulatory techniques, myofascial release, and counterstrain focusing on the T10–T12 areas.
What osteopathic techniques may increase parasympathetic tone?	Muscle energy to the occipito-atlantal (OA), balance ligamentous tension, suboccipital release, OA decompression, and other techniques that can affect the vagus nerve.

235

What osteopathic techniques are contraindicated in the postoperative patient?

High velocity low amplitude.

THIRD SPACING

What are the signs of third spacing?

Tachycardia, edema (especially in the extremities), and decreased urine output.

When does third-spaced fluid mobilize back into the intravascular space?

Usually around the third postoperative day.

How can third spacing be managed using osteopathic manipulation?

Lymphatic techniques.

What is necessary before performing any lymphatic treatment?

Release of all diaphragms en route for lymph return to the thoracic duct.

List the major contraindications to lymphatic treatment.

Fractures, severe infections (temperature > 102°F), abscess, carcinoma.*

*The contraindication to lymphatic treatment in carcinoma is controversial.

CHAPTER 20 EMERGENCY MEDICINE

THE ACUTE CARDIAC PATIENT

What is the first-line treatment for an acute myocardial infarction (MI)?	**The first-line treatment for MI continues to be O$_2$, nitroglycerin, aspirin, morphine, heparin, β-blocker, and ACE inhibitor.**
What is the utility of OMT in an acute MI?	OMT can help to normalize the significant autonomic imbalances that present within 30 minutes post-MI, leading to significant reductions in complications and mortality. *Note: similar rational for early initiation of β-blockers in MI.*
When is OMT indicated in acute MI?	Only after the patient has been stabilized and pharmacologic management initiated. "Time is myocardium," and because OMT can augment autonomic benefits of medications to prevent further ischemic changes, it can be used in the ED.
How soon after an MI do afferent reflexes occur?	Within a few seconds of an infarction, cardio-cardiac reflexes can predispose one to ventricular arrhythmias.
What is the danger of increased sympathetic nervous system (SNS) tone in an MI?	Increased SNS tone can lead to generation of ectopic foci, arrhythmias, and inhibit collateral circulation. It may also cause coronary vasoconstriction, increased heart rate, and increased total peripheral resistance. Thus, increasing afterload and O$_2$ demand causing further ischemia and reducing myocardial recovery.
What are the effects of excessive parasympathetic nervous system (PNS) tone in MI patients?	Excessive PNS stimulation may lead to bradyarrhythmias, hypotension, decreased coronary perfusion, and therefore more ischemia.
What techniques should be used in acute MI?	**Indirect or soft tissue techniques addressing the SNS and PNS innervation to the heart, fascial connections to the heart (from sternum, hyoid, and diaphragm), and lymphatic techniques such as pectoral traction.**

How can bradycardia be treated with OMT in the acute setting?	Because the right vagus nerve innervates the sinoatrial (SA) node, treating dysfunctions in the right occipito-atlantal (OA), atlanto-axial (AA), and OM suture can decrease PNS tone and treat bradyarrhythmias. *Note: similar rational for giving atropine to lower vagal tone.*
How can OMT be used to treat heart blocks in the ED?	The left vagus gives the major input of fibers supplying the AV node, where hyperstimulation may cause decreased electrical conduction. Therefore, treatments directed to the left OA, AA, and OM suture might normalize the vagal influences.
What is the application of OMM in emergent supraventricular tachycardia (SVT)?	Treatment of the right SNS fibers (T1 to T6) can decrease SNS input to the SA node thus, and decrease the generation of SVT.
Are there any trigger-points that may be treated to terminate SVT?	Treating the pectoralis trigger-point (right fifth intercostal space near right sternal border) has been shown to end SVT.

THE ACUTE RESPIRATORY PATIENT

What is the advantage of treating acute asthma/chronic obstructive pulmonary disease (COPD) with OMT in the ED?	OMT in conjunction with pharmacologic therapy can decrease hospital admission rates, length of hospital stay, and the number and dosages of drugs required to relieve symptoms of exacerbations.
What somatic dysfunctions are typically seen in patients with cough?	Coughing causes rapid contraction of the intercostal muscles, which may cause exhalation rib somatic dysfunctions.
What somatic dysfunctions are often found in obstructive pulmonary patients?	**Air trapping and hyperinflation of the lungs leads to flattening of the diaphragm, and inhalation dysfunctions of the ribs, especially ribs 3 and 4 on the left.**
What are less common somatic dysfunctions that are seen in severe COPD?	Exhalation somatic dysfunctions of ribs 1 and 2 (which are relatively uncommon somatic dysfunctions) can be seen in severe exacerbations of COPD when there is fatigue of the scalene muscles.

How can manipulation of the thoracic cage be used to treat acute respiratory distress?	OMT directed at the thoracic cage can increase tidal volume by up to 400 cc for each 1-cm increase in thoracic diameter. This can lead to increased aeration of underventilated regions in the lung, thereby leading to improvement in lung ventilation-to-perfusion ratio (V/Q) and improvement in respiratory function (pCO_2, O_2 saturation, total lung capacity, and residual volume).
When is the appropriate time to institute OMT in a patient in acute respiratory distress?	**OMT may be initiated in the ED simultaneously with pharmacologic therapy (i.e., receiving nebulizer treatments).**
What cranial somatic dysfunction is frequently associated with asthma?	**Extension dysfunction of the sphenobasilar synchondrosis (SBS).**
What is the role of treating the SNS in acute respiratory distress?	Stimulation of sympathetic nerves causes bronchodilation of the respiratory tree and increased ventilation. *Note: similar rationale for using inhaled β-agonists.*
What disturbance of the PNS is seen in obstructive pulmonary disease?	Asthma/COPD patients often have increased vagal tone that can cause bronchoconstriction, air trapping, and obstructive pathology.
What is the SNS innervation to the lungs?	**T1–T6, especially T3 and T4 on the left.**
What somatic dysfunctions are associated with heightened vagal tone?	**OM, OA, AA, C_2 restrictions.**
How are the treatment goals in acute respiratory distress different than in chronic treatments?	Whereas chronic treatment focuses on decreased exacerbations and trigger avoidance, acute management should be directed at increasing SNS stimulation, decreasing chest wall resistance, increasing thoracic diameter, and inhibiting vagal tone to improve oxygenation and ventilation immediately.
What special care must be taken when performing OMT on the acute respiratory patient?	Acute patients often are not comfortable lying down and need to be treated sitting up.
What techniques can be used to stimulate the SNS in a seated patient?	Seated rib-raising techniques and springing the angles of the ribs (with the thenar eminence) may be used to release restrictions of the ribs on the sympathetic ganglia.

Can cranial techniques be used in acute respiratory distress?	Yes, some authorities recommend starting the treatment of a patient in respiratory distress with a CV_4 to treat the extension somatic dysfunction of the SBS. This may be done seated if the patient is unable to lie down.

THE ACUTE TRAUMA PATIENT

Can OMT be used to treat acute trauma patients in the ED?	**OMT may be used in the initial presentation of trauma patients in the ED as long as the patient is hemodynamically stable, fractures have been ruled out, and neurovascular function has been assessed and is intact.**
What are the immediate advantages of treating acute trauma patients with OMT?	Those treated with OMT have shown significant decreases in pain and edema immediately after receiving OMT in the ED.
What benefits of early OMT in trauma patients were seen at short-term follow-up?	At 1-week follow-up trauma patients who were initially treated with OMT in the ED showed significant increases in range of motion versus patients not receiving OMT.
What potential problems can be avoided with OMT added in the early treatment of trauma?	OMT may help to decrease or avoid chronic pain, mobility and range of motion restriction, and other consequences of long-standing somatic dysfunctions.

21 ORTHOPEDIC SURGERY

SPINE: HERNIATED DISCS

What is a herniated disc?	The nucleus pulposus of the intervertebral disc protrudes through the annulus fibrosus.
In what direction does nucleus pulposus herniation occur and why?	Posterolateral herniation is most common because the posterior longitudinal ligament is weakest just lateral to the midline.
What intervertebral discs are most commonly herniated?	L_4–L_5 (compressing the L5 spinal nerve root) and L_5–S_1 (compressing the S1 spinal nerve root) account for 95% of disk herniations in the lumbar area. C_5–C_6 (compressing the C6 spinal nerve root) and C_6–C_7 (compressing the C7 spinal nerve root) account for the majority in the cervical area.
What special tests would be used to diagnose a herniated disc in the lumbar area?	Lumbar list test: patient standing, check for truncal shift to one side. Flip sign: patient seated, extension of the spine and pain when the leg is flexed at the hip. Femoral stretch test: patient prone; pain with hip extension. Straight leg test: Same as flip test except patient is supine and the leg to be tested is raised straight.
What special tests would be used to diagnose a herniated disc in the cervical area?	Spurling maneuver, axial compression, and Valsalva maneuver can illicit pain and/or radicular symptoms if positive result. Axial distraction test result is positive if pain decreases. *See Chapter 3: Cervical—Special Tests for details on these tests.*
What treatment modalities are usually used with herniated discs?	Conservative treatment initially, consisting of rest, immobilization, NSAIDs and OMT, because patients usually do well without surgical intervention.

What OMM treatment could be used?	Once the acute symptoms have subsided, discogenic facilitated positional release may be very useful in treatment. Balanced ligamentous tension (BLT), muscle energy (ME), myofascial release, or high velocity low amplitude, can be used by an experienced practitioner.

UPPER EXTREMITY: ACROMIOCLAVICULAR SEPARATION

What is the most common mechanism for an acromioclavicular (AC) separation?	Direct trauma from a fall on the "point" (acromion process) of the shoulder.
What structures serve as the major attachments of the clavicle to the scapula?	AC and coracoclavicular (CC) ligaments. The CC has two parts: conoid and trapezoid.
How do you classify/grade AC separations?	They are graded I–VI I: AC capsule sprain, no damage to CC II: AC capsule torn, sprained CC III: Complete tear of AC and CC ligament = separation of joint and instability. IV, V, and VI: Uncommon; involve position of clavicle in relation to the acromion. IV—posterior, V—superior, VI—inferior
What are the treatments for the different grades of AC separation?	Grades I and II: Conservative management, including OMT and sling. Grades IV, V, VI: Surgical repair Grade III: Controversial, dependent on patient's pain tolerance and preference.

UPPER EXTREMITY: SHOULDER INJURIES

What changes in the glenohumeral joint lead to an impingement syndrome and eventually to a tear of the rotator cuff?	Repetitive overhead motion (throwing) or degenerative changes fray the subacromial bursa. The resulting increased pressure on the rotator cuff tendons (most commonly supraspinatus tendon) is known as impingement syndrome. This causes the tendons to wear away due to increased friction against the acromion process.

What special tests can be used to diagnose rotator cuff pathology?	Neer impingement sign—With the scapula stabilized, raise patient's arm overhead in the sagittal plane. Positive test result will result in pain due to subacromial impingement.
	Hawkins sign—Forward flex arm to 90 degrees, flex elbow to 90 degrees, then internally rotate (IR) and look for pain.
	Empty can test: Bilaterally abduct arms to 90 degrees and then IR. Ask patient to resist downward force. Positive test result = pain or weakness indicating rotator cuff (supraspinatus) tear or impingement. Also known as the supraspinatus test.
What is the main determinant of stability of the glenohumeral joint?	**The soft tissue glenohumeral capsule surrounding the joint.**
What structures reinforce the glenohumeral capsule?	Superior, middle, and inferior (anterior and posterior bands) glenohumeral ligaments.
What is the most common type of shoulder dislocation?	Anterior or anterior/inferior (subcoracoid) dislocation of the humeral head.
What special tests can be used to detect a subcoracoid dislocation of the shoulder?	Apprehension test: abduction and external rotation of patient's arm reproduces pain and feeling that "shoulder will slip out of joint."
	Sulcus sign: put patient's arm to side, apply downward traction. Increased space in acromiohumeral sulcus signifies instability.
What is the most common cause of an anterior dislocation of the shoulder?	**Trauma when the shoulder is abducted and externally rotated. The subscapularis tendon moves away from anterior joint capsule with external rotation and abduction, exposing the anterior capsule and weakening the protective anterior joint structures.**
How does the patient with an anterior shoulder dislocation present?	**Patient's arm at their side, flattening of the once round contour of the shoulder, anterior prominence (the humeral head), and, in 10% of patients, axillary nerve damage (deltoid numbness).**
How could OMM be used in an anterior shoulder dislocation?	Post-reduction, once acute signs and symptoms have subsided and the patient is fully healed, rehab of the shoulder using the Spencer technique to facilitate range of motion.

What are other indications for the Spencer maneuver/treatment protocol?	• Postoperative rehabilitation of any surgical procedure of the shoulder • Adhesive capsulitis • Post-reduction of dislocated shoulder • Restoring range of motion in a patient with a rotator cuff tear or AC separation once the acute signs and symptoms subside and the injury is healed.
What are the contraindications for the Spencer technique?	Acute trauma, chronic glenohumeral instability, acute partial/full thickness rotator cuff tear.

LOWER EXTREMITY: HIP FRACTURES

What is the most common location of hip fracture?	Fracture of the femoral neck proximal to the intertrochanteric line or at the level of the intertrochanteric line.
In what population is a hip fracture most likely to occur?	**Geriatric population, age is the number-1 risk factor for hip fractures due to the increased prevalence of osteoporosis.**
How does a patient with a hip fracture usually present?	Lying down, with the affected leg in external rotation (due to gluteus maximus, piriformis mm.), abducted (due to gluteus maximus m.), and slightly shorter in length (due to iliopsoas m.).

LOWER EXTREMITY: ANTERIOR CRUCIATE LIGAMENT INJURIES

What is the function of the anterior cruciate ligament (ACL)?	Provides rotatory stability to the knee and prevents anterior translation (slide) of the tibia on the femur.
What is the most common mechanism for ACL tears?	A twisting or pivoting non-contact injury that may be accompanied by an audible "pop."
What special test(s) can be used to check for ACL pathology?	Lachman's test: knee in 20 to 30 degrees flexion. Examiner places one hand behind knee (proximal tibia) and the other on the distal thigh. The proximal tibia is pulled anteriorly with the hand behind the knee while the thigh is stabilized. Increased anterior translation of the tibia without a firm endpoint is a positive test result. Anterior drawer test: Similar to above, however the knee is flexed to 90 degrees.

Pivot shift test: With patient supine and completely relaxed, examiner supports the patient's leg behind the knee and at the ankle. Knee is flexed 20 to 30 degrees. If ACL is torn, the femur will drop backward (tibia subluxes anteriorly). Then examiner places knee in full extension while applying valgus stress and IR. The posterior capsule of the knee will reduce the subluxation, causing a snapping motion, indicative of a positive test result.

Alternatively, a positive test result may also result from reduction with flexion of the knee (40 degrees) due to the iliotibial band.

What is the conservative treatment for ACL injuries?	**Strengthening the hamstring mm. prevents anterior translation of the tibia, thus compensating for any ACL deficit.**

LOWER EXTREMITY: MENISCAL INJURIES

What is the most common mechanism of tears of the medial and/or lateral menisci?	Younger patient: a twisting injury. Older patient: degenerative changes.
What are the most common complaints of a patient with a torn meniscus?	Knee stiffness and a locking, popping, or clicking sound/feel. Patient will also feel pain when trying to squat.
What are the initial tests for meniscal damage?	Pain in joint line at the respective collateral ligament. McMurray's test: patient supine, flex knee, then internal (or external) rotation of the tibia and extension of knee while applying valgus force. Audible snap or click upon extension indicates possible tear of medial meniscus (lateral meniscus).

LOWER EXTREMITY: ANKLE SPRAIN

What is the most common kind of ankle sprain?	A sprain of the lateral ligament complex due to a forceful inversion injury.
What ligaments make up the lateral ligament complex?	Anterior talofibular ligament, posterior talofibular ligament, calcaneofibular ligaments.
Which of the three lateral complex ligaments is usually torn?	Anterior <u>TaloF</u>ibular ligament.  *Memory Aid:* <u>ATF</u>—<u>A</u>lways <u>T</u>ears <u>F</u>irst The calcaneofibular ligament is the second most commonly torn.

What is the most common mechanism of a sprain of the medial ankle ligament(s)?	A forceful eversion injury.
What medial ligament of the ankle is most commonly damaged?	Deltoid ligament.
What kind of fracture usually occurs with an eversion sprain due to the strong deltoid ligament?	Avulsion fracture of the medial malleolus. The superior fibers of the deltoid ligament attach to the inferior aspect of the medial malleolus.
What OMT can be used to treat an ankle sprain?	Once the acute pain subsides, any lymphatic drainage technique (ankle effleurage) can decrease the swelling at the ankle. Soft tissue techniques including BLT, ligamentous articular strain, and counterstrain are effective in improving long-term results after sprains.

LOWER EXTREMITY: ACHILLES TENDONITIS/RUPTURE

What is Achilles tendonitis?	Inflammation of the Achilles tendon, usually due to overuse, that most commonly causes pain near its insertion on the posterior aspect of the calcaneus.
The tendons of what muscles comprise the Achilles tendon?	**Gastrocnemius and soleus mm.**
What is the most common mechanism for an Achilles tendon rupture?	Forceful plantar-flexion injury: patients report hearing a pop and experiencing immediate severe calf pain.
What signs and symptoms will a patient with a ruptured Achilles tendon report?	Inability to push off with the affected foot as they walk and instability when placing any stress on the affected side. This is because the two muscles that make up the Achilles tendon are responsible for plantar flexion and stabilizing the ankle joint.
What test is performed to assess the integrity of the Achilles tendon?	**Thompson test: Patient is prone or kneeling on a chair with their knee flexed to 90 degrees. In a positive test result, there will be an absence of the normal plantar flexion response of the foot to the calf squeezing.**
Which OMM techniques can strengthen the Achilles tendon?	**ME of the ankle using both plantarflexion and dorsiflexion maneuvers.**

CHAPTER 22 UROLOGY

URINARY TRACT INFECTION

What vertebral levels are the kidneys located in the recumbent position?	T_{12}–L_3 (the left kidney is usually half a vertebra higher than the right).
What is the lymphatic drainage of the kidneys?	Lymphatic vessels follow the renal vein to the lumbar (aortic) lymph nodes, which drain into the cisterna chyli.
What are the autonomics to the kidney?	**Sympathetic nervous innervation in the spinal cord at the level of T10–T11. Parasympathetic innervation arises from the vagus nerve.**
List the congenital anomalies of the lower urinary tract that predispose to urinary tract infections (UTIs).	Extrophy, epispadias, patent urachus, posterior urethral valves, and cryptorchidism.
What physical findings would support a diagnosis of a UTI?	↑ frequency/urgency/pain with urination; costovertebral angle tenderness, Chapman's reflexes, collateral ganglion involvement, and the pattern of segmental somatic dysfunction.
When will Lloyd's punch test be positive?	Kidney infection and/or posterior peritoneal irritation.
What are the osteopathic considerations in patients with dysuria and frequency?	**Ruling out pubic symphyseal and pelvic floor somatic dysfunctions.**
What are the goals of osteopathic treatment of UTIs?	Treatment of pelvic floor somatic dysfunction to improve symptomatology and help relieve prostatic congestion. Treat trigger points as they can also cause urinary frequency, urgency, sphincter spasm, residual urine, or bladder pain.
What are the Chapman's points of the kidneys and bladder?	**Chapman's points to the kidneys are located on the ipsilateral side, one-inch lateral and one-inch superior to the umbilicus. Anterior Chapman's viscerosomatic reflexes for the bladder are located periumbilically.** *See Figure 1.1 on Chapman's points.*

What factors increase the risk of an ascending UTI?	Incomplete bladder emptying, reflux and loss of normal ureteral peristalsis.
How can UTIs be treated with OMT?	**Normalize the sympathetic activity at T10–L2, the parasympathetics from the vagus nerve proximally, and S2–S4 distally. Improve lymphatic drainage to the area in order to reduce congestion and improve tissue defense.**
How can faulty posture and nephroptosis (drooping of the kidney) increase urologic disease in a patient?	The slumped thorax increases downward pressure onto the kidneys, which decreases the protecting fat layer. This leads to chronic passive congestion, kinked ureters, hydronephrosis, orthostatic albuminuria, urinary stasis, stones, and infection.

URETEROLITHIASIS

What are the common causes of ureteral irritation?	Ureterolithiasis, ureterospasms, appendicitis, and psoas abscess/spasm.
Where is pain from ureteral distention referred?	Upper ureter (T10–T12) pain refers to the anterior superior iliac spine, lateral to the border of the rectus abdominis muscle.
	Middle ureter (T11–L1) pain refers to the inguinal ligament anterior to the rectus abdominis muscle.
	Lower ureter (T12–L2) pain refers to the suprapubic area and into the scrotum or labia.
Which five regions of the ureter are most vulnerable to obstruction from a calculus?	1. Ureteropelvic junction
	2. External iliac vessels at the pelvic brim
	3. Juxtaposition between vas deferens and ureters
	4. As the ureter angulates anteromedially
	5. Ureterovesical junction.
What musculoskeletal finding is commonly found with ureteral dysfunction?	**Psoas dysfunction presenting as a psoatic gait. The patient may stand with hip and knee flexed due to associated psoas spasm.**
What is the osteopathic treatment protocol for ureteral irritation?	Normalizing the sympathetics (to reduce ureterospasm) with thoracolumbar paraspinal inhibition and/or gentle rib raising.
	Using counterstrain treatment of palpable myofascial tender points.

Assuring adequate lymphatic drainage to prevent complications and tissue damage.

Treating psoas spasm, which can cause ureteral dysfunction.

PROSTATITIS

What is the lymphatic drainage of the prostate gland?	Lymphatic drainage from the prostate gland is to the internal iliac and sacral lymph nodes.
What is the innervation to the prostate gland?	**Parasympathetics: pelvic splanchnic nerves (S2–S4).** **Sympathetics: inferior hypogastric plexus (L1, L2).**
What are the symptoms of acute prostatitis?	Fever, chills, myalgia, arthralgia, perineal/low-back pain, decreased urinary stream, and terminal dribbling.
What are the signs of acute prostatitis?	Gross hematuria; tender, warm, and swollen prostate gland.
What effect does sympathetic nervous system have on the prostate gland?	Sympathetics via the hypogastric nerves (T10 or T12 through L2) causes the smooth muscle in the walls of the prostate to contract and force secretions into the urethra during ejaculation.
What are the goals of OMT in the treatment of acute prostatitis?	Along with antibiotics, treating the ischiorectal fossa T10–L2 (sympathetics) and S2–S4 (parasympathetics) helps maximize prostatic levels of antibiotics and assists the body's natural defenses.
Where are Chapman's points referring to the prostate gland?	**Myofascial tissues along the posterior margin of the iliotibial band.** *See Figure 1.1 on Chapman's points.*

URINARY INCONTINENCE

What is the parasympathetic innervation to the bladder?	**S2–S4 (via the pelvic splanchnic nerves and hypogastric plexus).**
What are the effects of parasympathetic innervation to the bladder?	Excitatory innervation to the detrusor muscle and inhibitory innervation to the trigone m.
What is the source of sympathetic innervation of the urinary bladder?	**T12–L2 to the sympathetic chain ganglia, the lumbar and sacral splanchnic nerve, and the inferior hypogastric plexus.**

What are the effects of sympathetic innervation to the bladder?	The trigone, which has alpha-adrenoceptors, contracts with sympathetic stimulation; while the detrusor m., which has beta-adrenoceptors, relaxes with stimulation. Both are necessary to allow bladder expansion while it fills.
For proper micturition, what three components have to be normal?	1. Excitation of the parasympathetic system to activate the detrusor muscle 2. Inhibition of the sympathetic system to relax the trigone and internal sphincter muscle 3. Subsequent inhibition of the pudendal nerve to relax the external urethra (sphincter) muscle.
What are the different types of incontinence?	• Urge: ~65% women (most common) • Stress: ~15% women • Overflow: ~10% • Functional: ~10% (patients can't get to bathroom in time).
What is urge urinary incontinence?	Unstable/overactive bladder (detrusor instability) with uninhibited bladder contractions. Patient has the sudden urge to void but does not make it to the bathroom in time.
What is the goal of OMT in urge urinary incontinence?	**To aid in bladder relaxation by treating facilitations of the sympathetics and parasympathetics in conjunction with anticholinergics.**
How can OMT address the sympathetics in the treatment of urge incontinence?	**Rib raising and balanced ligamentous tension to T10–L2 region; Chapman's reflexes of the bladder (anterior and midline in the umbilical area between L3–L4); inferior mesenteric ganglion release.**
How can OMT address the parasympathetics in the treatment of urge incontinence?	**Pelvic rock to treat somatic dysfunction in the sacrum and sacroiliac joints to normalize parasympathetic innervation from the pelvic splanchnic nerves (S2–S4).**
What is stress urinary incontinence?	Incontinence with coughing, laughing, sneezing, lifting heavy objects due to weakened pelvic floor mm. and/or urethral incompetence.
How do Kegel exercises help with stress urinary incontinence?	Kegel exercises strengthen the levator ani and coccygeus mm., which support the urethra, bladder, uterus, and rectum.

What is overflow incontinence?	Diminished stream and leakage of small amounts of urine with a large residual volume in the bladder.
What can cause overflow incontinence?	• Benign prostatic hypertrophy (BPH) or a urethral stricture • Neurogenic bladder most likely with diabetes mellitus • Overuse of anticholinergic drugs.
How can overflow incontinence be treated?	Depending on the etiology: • Abstain from anticholinergic medications • Bladder outflow obstruction and BPH medication • Transurethral resection of the prostate (T. U. R. P.) • Foley catheterization (indwelling or intermittent).

SEXUAL DYSFUNCTION

What does proper sexual functioning involve?	Interaction of somatic, parasympathetic, and sympathetic reflexes with cortical factors.
What is the autonomic nervous system involvement in ejaculation?	The lumbar splanchnic nn. via the hypogastric n. to the vas deferens, seminal vesicles, prostate and internal urethral sphincter. This is aided by somatic influence from sacral plexus, via the pudendal n. to the bulbospongiosis m.
Which osteopathic findings must be addressed in sexual dysfunction?	Restrictions over the inferior mesenteric ganglion and facilitations at T_{10}–L_2 vertebral and paraspinal regions.
What are the goals of OMT in erectile dysfunction?	**Decrease sacroiliac somatic dysfunction to address the somatic innervation (via the pudendal n.) and the parasympathetic reflexes (S2–S4) in erectile dysfunction.** **The somatic dysfunctions/facilitations from the sympathetic innervation (T10–T11) must also be addressed.**

CHAPTER 23 RADIOLOGY

INTRODUCTION TO READING RADIOGRAPHS

What are the preliminary items to note when approaching a plain or axial film?

First: Identify patient name, medical record number, age and sex, check if previous studies exist for comparison, plane of study, quality, and region being examined.

Then: Read film with a systematic and orderly approach.

What qualifies as an adequate chest radiograph (CXR)?

1. Rotation: Medial part of clavicle equidistant from spine.
2. Inspiration: Diaphragm located at or below posterior rib 10 and anterior rib 8.
3. Exposure: Bronchovascular markings are seen adequately in lungs and through the heart.

What are the relative differences between a posteroanterior (PA) and an anteroposterior (AP) view on a plain CXR?

AP or portable films: Heart appears larger, the posterior ribs appear more horizontal.

PA films: Heart borders are sharp and distinct, heart size representative of actual size and scapulae are retracted.

Describe the "ABCDE" systematic approach to a plain CXR.

Alignment: Trachea, aorta, and mediastinum.

Bones and **B**orders: Ribs, clavicles, scapulae, humeri, sternum, vertebral bodies, pleura.

Cardiac: Position, silhouette, $<\frac{1}{2}$ size of chest, calcifications.

Diaphragm: Elevation, depression, costophrenic angles, adjacent abdominal structures.

Extent of field: Soft tissue, vascularity, gross abnormalities.

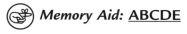 *Memory Aid:* **ABCDE**

What are the radiographic requirements in evaluating a fracture?

The fracture line must be demonstrated in two or more views. Radiographic studies of 1 joint above and below must be performed.

COMMON RADIOLOGIC STUDIES

What are the advantages and disadvantages of a plain radiograph?	**Advantage: Quick initial assessment, inexpensive, primarily used for evaluating bony deformities, abdominal opacities, air-fluid levels, free air, etc.** **Disadvantage: Radiation, poor soft tissue and organ visualization.**
What are the advantages and disadvantages of a CT?	**Advantage: Fast, used in acute trauma, bony detail.** **Disadvantage: Radiation, contrast use (contraindicated in renal failure), and cost.**
What are the advantages and disadvantages of an MRI?	Advantage: No radiation, multi-plane imaging, soft tissue details. Disadvantage: Slow, contraindications (metal objects, pacemaker), and cost.
What are the advantages and disadvantages of ultrasound (US)?	Advantage: Noninvasive, for severely ill, differentiates cystic vs. solid, guidance for biopsy. Disadvantage: Operator-dependent, some substances compromise image quality (i.e., air, bone, and barium).

AXIAL COLUMN

A 39-year-old woman with pain and paresthesia also has cyanotic episodes at the neck, shoulder, and upper extremity. No cervical rib is palpable and the Spurling maneuver is negative. Thoracic inlet syndrome is suspected. What radiologic and osteopathic findings may be present?	CXR/CT: Evaluates the anatomy for causes of impingement, presence of anomalies, and disease processes (e.g., fractures, neoplasms). OMT: Rib 1 elevated, superiorly rotated clavicle, Sibson's fascial restriction, and anterior and middle scalene mm. hypertonicity.
How is scoliosis diagnosed?	**XR: Spinal elements are laterally deviated, forming a convexity. The Cobb angle can be measured on an AP film of the spine.** *See Chapter 4: Thoracic—Clinical Anatomy for information on Cobb Angle.* **OMT: Spinal segments are rotated and sidebent to opposite sides (type I group curve), paravertebral muscle spasm (PVMS) on convex side, leg length discrepancy, and whole body compensation.**

A 45-year-old man has lower back pain (LBP) that radiates down to his toe. Pain began suddenly while moving furniture. The straight leg raise test is positive. Lumbar PVMS is noted with restrictions of L_4 and L_5. A herniated disc at the L_4–L_5 interspace is suspected. What is the radiological test of choice and preferred osteopathic treatment?

MRI (TOC): Disc bulge, vertebral degeneration, spinal cord and nerve root impingement, and stenosis.

OMT: Lumbar discogenic facilitated positional release is the osteopathic treatment of choice. May also use myofascial, muscle energy, balanced ligamentous tension, counterstrain, and high velocity low amplitude in the hands of an experienced physician.

What is a Scotty Dog sign?

An anatomic landmark outlined by the vertebral spine, seen in oblique radiographs of the spine.

What are the anatomic landmarks of a Scotty Dog?

Ear/tail: Superior articular processes

Nose: Transverse process (TP)

Eye: Pedicle

Legs: Inferior articular processes

Neck: Pars-interarticularis.

How is a spondylolysis diagnosed?

Oblique XR: Detects a pars-interarticularis defect visualized as an imaginary "collar" at the neck of the Scotty Dog.

How is spondylolisthesis diagnosed?

Lateral and oblique XR: Anterior slippage of a vertebral body above relative to the one below, with disc space narrowing and osteophyte formation.

A 30-year-old man with history of rheumatologic disease and (+)HLA-B27 presents with LBP and limited motion at the waist. Patient is unable to sidebend and flex at the lumbar spine. An AP radiograph of the lumbar and sacrum shows a bamboo spine (Figure 23.1). What is the diagnosis?

Dx: Ankylosing spondylitis

XR: Sacroiliitis, narrow sacroiliac joint, fusion of vertebral bodies (bamboo spine), degenerative vertebral changes.

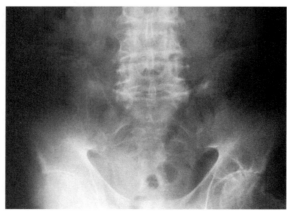

FIGURE 23.1 – Bamboo spine.

UPPER EXTREMITY

What XR views are required to diagnose an anterior dislocation of the shoulder?

AP XR with internal and external rotation, and a transaxillary (scapular-Y) view to assess humeral head location.

How is a rotator cuff or supraspinatus tear diagnosed with radiologic imaging?

MRI (TOC): Evaluates the tear, which is located primarily at the superior aspect of the glenoid labrum.

XR: Shows narrowing of the acromial-humeral space with erosions and cortical changes of the humeral head.

A 24-year-old man complains of left wrist pain after falling on his outstretched hand while playing basketball. On physical examination, mild swelling is noted at the lateral wrist. Palpatory and motion testing of the carpal bones reveals severe tenderness over the scaphoid, no bone dislocations (Figure 23.2). What is the diagnosis?

Dx: Scaphoid fracture

XR (TOC): Can be negative in acute phase. Possible development of avascular necrosis is indicated by increased density at the proximal pole of the scaphoid.

MRI/Bone Scan: Definitive diagnosis.

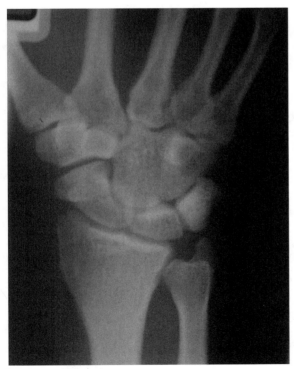

FIGURE 23.2 – Wrist pain.

LOWER EXTREMITY

A 78-year-old woman complains of left hip pain and inability to walk after a fall. Upon initial examination, the left hip appears shorter and externally rotated (Figure 23.3). What is the diagnosis?

Dx: Left femoral neck fracture

XR: Shows fracture line through the femur. Must r/o displacement of femoral head with lateral view film.

CT/MRI/Bone Scan: r/o the possibility of a pathologic fracture.

OMT: Contraindicated!

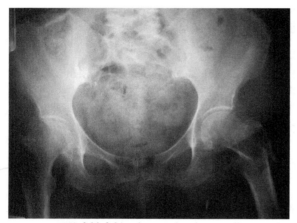

FIGURE 23.3 – Painful left hip, shortened and externally rotated.

A 14-year-old obese boy complains of left hip and knee pain of gradual onset. Patient is observed to have an antalgic gait. A lateral frog-leg radiograph of the left hip is shown (Figure 23.4). What is the diagnosis?

Dx: Slipped capital femoral epiphysis (SCFE)

XR (AP and frog-legged lateral): Femoral head (ice cream scoop) appears to be slipping off of femoral neck (cone). There is slight widening of the physis and blanching of metaphysis.

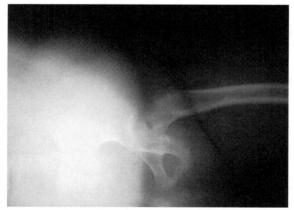

FIGURE 23.4 – Scoop of ice cream (femoral head) slipping off of a cone (femoral neck).

CHEST

A 53-year-old man presents with productive cough, fever, chills, dyspnea, and chest pain. A diagnosis of bacterial pneumonia is made. What are the radiographic and correlated osteopathic findings?

CXR (TOC): Patchy opacity that can progress to lobar consolidation.

OMT: Viscerosomatic reflexes of parasympathetic nervous system (PNS) at OA and sympathetic nervous system (SNS) at T_1–T_6, thoracic aperture and diaphragm restrictions. Warmth or tactile fremitus at area of consolidation.

A 46-year-old man with progressive dyspnea and abnormal pulmonary function test results is diagnosed with emphysema. What are the radiographic and correlated osteopathic findings?

CXR: Hyperinflation with flat/serrated diaphragm, decreased vascular markings, bullous changes.

OMT: Viscerosomatic reflexes of PNS at OA and SNS at T_1–T_6, and thoracic aperture, diaphragm, and accessory muscles restrictions (sternocleidomastoid, scalenes, serratus anterior, etc.).

A 71-year-old woman presents with exertional and paroxysmal nocturnal dyspnea, orthopnea, 2+ pitting edema, S_3 gallop, and crackles. With a diagnosis of congestive heart failure (CHF), what are the expected radiologic (CXR and echocardiogram) and correlated osteopathic findings?

CXR: Kerley B-lines, cardiomegaly, effusions ("bat's wing" pattern) and cephalization.

Echocardiogram: Enlarged left ventricle, low ejection fraction, and valvular incompetence.

OMT: Viscerosomatic reflexes of PNS at OA and SNS at T_1–T_4, restricted thoracic aperture and diaphragm, with widespread edema located primarily in dependent areas (lower extremity).

After three unsuccessful attempts for central venous catheterization (via the right subclavian v.), a 60-year-old male patient complains of shortness of breath (SOB) and difficulty breathing. Physical exam demonstrates decreased breath sounds and rib movement on the right. A stat portable film (Figure 23.5) is ordered. What is the diagnosis and how is it treated?

Diagnosis: Right apical pneumothorax

Treatment: Thoracostomy tube

See Chapter 5: Ribs—Clinical Anatomy for description of thoracostomy tube placement.

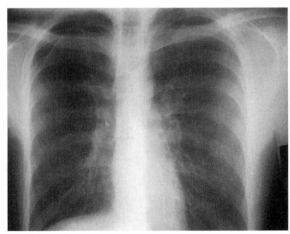

FIGURE 23.5 – Shortness of breath.

257

A 57-year-old diaphoretic man presents with SOB, crushing substernal chest pain radiating to his right arm. With a diagnosis of MI, what are the expected radiologic (angiogram, CXR, echocardiogram, and nuclear scan) and correlated osteopathic findings?

Angiography (TOC): Extent of stenosis.

CXR: Can show pulmonary edema and CHF secondary to papillary muscle rupture.

Echocardiogram: Noninvasive, detects papillary rupture and wall motion.

Nuclear "hot spots": areas of infarct that pick up the tracer.

OMT: Facilitated cord segments of PNS at the OA and SNS at T_1–T_4 on the left, trigger point at the anterior pectoralis mm. can cause tachyarrhythmias, and findings such as a flat curve or scoliosis can be a causal source.

Abdomen and Pelvis

A 45-year-old woman with nausea and vomiting, abdominal pain, and distention also has high-pitched bowel sounds. A diagnosis of small bowel obstruction is made. What radiologic (abdominal plain film, CT) and osteopathic findings are expected?

Abdominal XR (TOC): Multiple dilated loops of bowel with air-fluid levels on upright film.

CT: Same as previous, identify transition point, determines underlying cause.

OMT: Viscerosomatic reflexes of SNS at T_5–L_2 and the PNS at the OA and S_2–S_4 (depending on region of bowel affected), and intestinal peristalsis Chapman's point 2 inches below anterior superior iliac spine.

A 24-year-old woman with decreased appetite, a low-grade fever and leukocytosis, right lower quadrant (RLQ) pain, and peritoneal signs is suspected to have appendicitis. What radiologic (abdominal plain film, CT, US) and osteopathic findings are expected?

CT: Shows enlarged, dilated, thickened appendix with fat streaking and occasionally fecalith.

Abdominal XR: Calcified fecalith in the RLQ, focal ileus, loss of psoas shadow and flank line.

US: Commonly used in children and women.

OMT: T_{10}/T_{12} on the right, ipsilateral psoas mm. restriction and Chapman's points: anteriorly—tip of right 12th rib and posteriorly—TP of T_{11}.

A 35-year-old obese female presents with post-prandial right upper quadrant (RUQ) pain that is worse when she eats fast food. Cholecystitis is suspected. What are the radiologic TOC and structural findings?

US (TOC for any RUQ pain): Gallbladder wall thickening, pericholecystic fluid, biliary sludge, possible stones with acoustic shadowing.

OMT: Viscerosomatic reflexes of PNS at OA and SNS at T_5 to T_7 on the right.

A 42-year-old male chronic alcoholic with fever, nausea, vomiting, and severe epigastric pain. Lab tests show an increase in amylase and lipase. What is the most likely diagnosis? What radiologic studies should be performed? What osteopathic structural findings can be found?

Dx—Acute pancreatitis

CT (TOC): Diffuse enlargement of pancreas with fat streaking. May also find calcification, pseudocyst, necrosis, or abscess.

Abdominal XR: "Sentinel loop" or "cut-off sign"

OMT: Viscerosomatic reflexes of PNS at OA and SNS at T_7 on the right.

A 57-year-old man with history of renal calculi presents with severe dysuria and inguinal pain that radiates to his flank. What radiologic studies are necessary? What osteopathic findings are expected with recurrent urolithiasis?

KUB (TOC): Detects opacities in the urinary tract, dilated renal pelvis and proximal ureter (with IV contrast).

CT (TOC): Detects hydronephrosis or external compression, radio-opaque stones without contrast, radiolucent stones with IV contrast.

US: Detects radio-opaque and lucent stones, and ureteral dilatation.

OMT: Viscerosomatic reflexes of PNS at OA and S_2–S_4 and SNS at T_{10}–L_2, Chapman's point anteriorly at 1 inch lateral and superior to the umbilicus and posteriorly at the space between the TP of T_{12} and L_1.

Note: Page numbers with an *f* indicate figures; those with a *t* indicate tables; those with an *n* indicate footnotes.